EVALUATOR
COMPETENCIES

EVALUATOR COMPETENCIES

Standards for the Practice of Evaluation in Organizations

DARLENE F. RUSS-EFT, PH.D.
MARCIE J. BOBER, PH.D.
ILEANA DE LA TEJA, PH.D.
MARGUERITE FOXON, PH.D.
TIFFANY A. KOSZALKA, PH.D.

Foreword by
HALLIE PRESKILL, PH.D.
2007 PRESIDENT, AMERICAN EVALUATION
ASSOCIATION

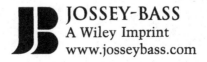

JOSSEY-BASS
A Wiley Imprint
www.josseybass.com

Published by Jossey-Bass
A Wiley Imprint
989 Market Street, San Francisco, CA 94103—www.josseybass.com

Jossey-Bass books and products are available through most bookstores. To contact Jossey-Bass directly call our Customer Care Department within the United States at (800) 956-7739, outside the United States at (317) 572-3986, or via fax at (317) 572-4002.

Jossey-Bass also publishes its books in a variety of electronic formats. Some content that appears in print may not be available in electronic books.

Library of Congress Cataloging-in-Publication Data

Evaluator competencies : standards for the practice of evaluation in organizations / Darlene F. Russ-Eft, . . . [et al.] ; foreword by Hallie Preskill. — 1st ed.
  p.   cm.—(Research methods for the social sciences)
  Includes bibliographical references.
  ISBN-13: 978-0-7879-9599-7 (cloth)
   1. Employees—Training of—Evaluation.   2. Personnel management—Evaluation.   3. Organizational learning—Evaluation.   4. Performance standards. I. Russ-Eft, Darlene F.
  HF5549.5.T7E894 2008
  658.3'124—dc22

                                                                            2007044997

FIRST EDITION

HB Printing   10 9 8 7 6 5 4 3 2 1

CONTENTS

PART TWO: THE IBSTPI EVALUATOR COMPETENCIES: VALIDATION

TABLES, EXHIBIT, AND FIGURES

TABLES

EXHIBIT

FIGURES

To Dennis Sheriff and George Pollard

Without your passionate belief in the vision of the Board, your commitments of time and energy, and your unfailing moral and financial support through the difficult years of the early 1990s, the Board would not have survived . . . nor these standards have been developed. Thank you!

FOREWORD

Can we afford *not* to evaluate? This is a question we learning and performance professionals need to ask of ourselves, our colleagues, and our organization's managers and leaders. At first blush, this question may seem flippant or even sarcastic. Yet, it is a question that is critically important to today's organizations especially for those in the training, learning, and performance fields. For decades now, human resource development (HRD) professionals have been struggling for respect, legitimacy, resources, and a voice and place at the strategic planning table. Although these professionals have increasingly been developing higher levels of knowledge and skills through various certificate and graduate education programs in adult learning, HRD, training, organization development, performance technology, and organizational psychology, they still tend to be more vulnerable to budget cuts; find their work being outsourced to others; and experience many obstacles when seeking support for conducting needs assessments, adequate time for designing and developing programs, and sufficient backing for ensuring learning transfer.

For many years, I have observed this situation and have come to believe that one major reason for the woes of HRD professionals is their lack of truly understanding the value of evaluation and how to conduct timely, useful, and credible evaluations of their programs, services, products, and systems. Although we can speculate on all of the reasons for this situation, I would argue that a significant reason is the field's failure to connect to the broader discipline and profession of evaluation. Trainers' over-reliance on Kirkpatrick's four-level evaluation approach has severely limited how trainers evaluate their programs, what they learn from their evaluations, and how credible and useful their evaluation results are judged by executives. Although the four levels certainly have some utility, it is nothing short of mind-boggling that the HRD field has not ventured beyond this approach (or variations on this approach) in the past 50 years. Until now. This book represents a major step forward for the training, learning, and performance field. It provides a valuable new lens for understanding the role of evaluation and the knowledge, skills, and attitudes necessary for ensuring that evaluation supports the work of HRD professionals and others committed to enhancing individual, group, and organizational learning. Perhaps it is no coincidence that this book is just becoming available at this particular moment in the profession's life cycle. As such, the following quote may be apropos: "Life is all about timing . . . the unreachable becomes reachable, the unavailable becomes available, the unattainable . . . attainable. Have the patience, wait it out. It's all about timing" (contemporary author, Stacey Charter). I believe that the HRD field is at the tipping point of what might be called the *evaluation imperative*. To this point, consider the following:

■ The American Society for Training and Development's 2005 State of the Industry report concluded that the organizations that received their BEST awards (awarded for demonstrating a clear link between learning and performance) were far more committed to and effective in evaluating the learning function's activities and impact.

■ A majority of job postings for trainers, performance technologists, learning specialists, and other HRD-related jobs are requiring applicants to have evaluation-related knowledge, skills, and experiences. It is no longer a nice-to-have but a need-to-have set of competencies.

■ The American Evaluation Association has more than 5,500 members who represent more than 75 countries and every sector of the economy. The annual conference, usually held in November, attracts approximately 2,500 attendees. The association's membership has grown more than 80 percent since 2001 and is growing at a rate of 10 to 15 percent per year.

■ There are now more than 75 regional and national evaluation associations, societies, and networks around the globe.

■ Organizations are increasingly collecting a variety of data on which to judge their performance and to be accountable to their stakeholders. Whether these are called learning analytics, metrics, dashboards, scorecards, or market research, there is mounting evidence that supports we are a data-driven society and that organizations want data to inform their decision-making processes.

The Evaluation Imperative is one that I have been committed to for nearly 30 years. As one who teaches graduate-level evaluation courses and conducts many evaluation workshops each year, I often begin by telling participants that I love evaluation. I tell them that evaluation is about learning, growth, and change. I tell them that evaluation is about asking questions, being curious, making decisions, and creating the future. And I tell them that I always get excited when starting a new evaluation project. Over the years, I have become accustomed to people's initial reactions, which are usually to think I am a little odd because they have rarely experienced evaluation in a way that reflects my passion. However, I have never been discouraged by their skeptical and sympathetic looks and comments because, in the end, my dedication to and enthusiasm for evaluation often rubs off on them, and much to their surprise, they develop an appreciation for the ways in which evaluation can contribute to their programs and organizations.

My passion for evaluation is rooted in one very simple conviction: that evaluation makes a difference. For it to make a difference, however, the evaluation's findings need to be used, and people must learn from the evaluation process and its outcomes. But regrettably, not everyone welcomes evaluation. In fact, many people view evaluation as punishing, threatening, mysterious, hurtful, and useless. So the question becomes, if we really want others to think evaluatively and use evaluation practices, then how can we help them reframe their perceptions of evaluation? I believe the answer is in helping people see the *possibilities* of evaluation.

Reframing our thinking about evaluation relates to reorienting how we see the world. For example, consider the following vignette as told by Rosamund and Benjamin Zander in their book, *The Art of Possibility*: "A shoe factory sends two marketing scouts to a region of Africa to study the prospects for expanding their business. One sends back a telegram saying, 'Situation hopeless. Stop. No one wears shoes.' The other writes back triumphantly, 'Glorious business opportunity. Stop. They have no shoes'" (p. 9). So which one represents possibilities? Which one reflects hope and optimism? For whom would you rather work? This anecdote leads me to wonder, how do we create a place where HRD professionals can see that evaluation is about creating possibilities—that is, possibilities for programs to be better, to be more, to be visible, to be known, and to make a difference?

Designing, conducting, and securing support for evaluations are not easy. As program evaluators, we often find ourselves in situations that require patience, political acumen, fortitude, resourcefulness, and diplomacy. But it is our commitment to evaluation, our belief in the possibilities of evaluation, and the value of evaluation that keep us going. Perhaps our biggest challenge as HRD evaluators is getting organization members to change their mental models of evaluation. That is, we need to help them perceive evaluation as something other than threatening, cumbersome, and useless. Instead, we should focus on enhancing organization members' ability to see the possibilities of evaluation so that they understand the value evaluation adds to the organization's vision and mission. Fortunately, this book contributes significantly to helping us think about, plan, and conduct effective evaluations: evaluations that ask the hard questions, that improve our practice, and that help us make better decisions about program purposes, priorities, resources, and approaches. The competencies described in this book reflect a broad range of evaluation concepts and practices that have been endorsed by the evaluation profession. Consequently, this book represents an important bridge for learning and performance professionals who desire to become more knowledgeable and skilled in evaluation and who wish to understand and communicate the value of evaluation to others. My hope is that after reading this book, your answer to the question, "Can we afford not to evaluate?" is a resounding "No! Let's get to it!"

Hallie Preskill, Ph.D.
2007 President, American Evaluation Association
School of Behavioral and Organizational Sciences
Claremont Graduate University

PREFACE

The International Board of Standards for Training, Performance, and Instruction (ibstpi®) embraces a mission to develop, validate, and promote the implementation of international standards to advance training, instruction, learning, and performance improvement for individuals and organizations. Within the mission of this professional service organization, 15 elected directors representing academic, corporate, government, and consulting agencies from around the world recognized a need for improving program evaluator performance. As such, the Evaluator Standards discussed in this book became the fourth in a series of standards of performance endorsed by ibstpi: Instructional Designer (2000), Training Manager (2001), Instructor (2003), and now Evaluator (2006). The three previous sets do include evaluation skills in the competencies; however, a comprehensive set of standards that focused on the foundations, planning and design, implementation, and management competencies of a professional evaluator did not yet exist. With evaluation gaining importance as a profession that is transdisciplinary and global, these standards were developed and validated to fill that void.

The development of ibstpi standards for improving performance is directed and informed by a 25-year history, the ibstpi competency development model, and the board's core values and guiding principles. For a history of ibstpi, see Appendix A.

The ibstpi competency development model, described later in this book, is a research-based development model that begins with job or role definition. It then blends research, practice, and a vision of the future with criticality data from professionals involved in evaluation, thus yielding competencies and performance statements with global relevance.

The board's core values include integrity, commitment to excellence, ethical practice, diverse perspectives, and collaboration. These values guide the principles of practice adopted by the directors: leadership by example, evidence-based decision making, collaborative development and implementation, global influence and relevance, continuous improvement, board continuity, service to the profession, and fiscal responsibility.

The values and guiding principles were exemplified in the development of the Evaluator Standards endorsed by the ibstpi directors. First, the process for validating these standards followed accepted legal and ethical practice that respects the privacy of people and organizations. The research protocols were established and approved within the guidelines of institutional review board requirements for the use of human participants. Next, diverse international perspectives were sought out and encouraged through director input and identifying and involving individuals and organizations around the world with experience in evaluation work. Third, evidence from the extensive worldwide validation study informed the final list of competencies and performance statements. Fourth, the directors collaborate on all projects but capitalize on the individual expertise to charge a subcommittee of directors who are recognized and respected leaders. In the case of the evaluator competencies, the project and subcommittee were led under the skillful direction of Drs. Darlene Russ-Eft and Marguerite Foxon, in collaboration with current and former directors, advisors, and fellows of the board. Their standing in the field made them the best choice for this project. Fifth, it is also important to underscore that those who direct the board's activities also strive for excellence in putting into practice the Evaluator Standards they endorse. The evaluation of board activities and workshops follows these standards and are guided by the evaluation experts on the board.

Consistent with its mission, the board commits at least three of its directors to "competency think tanks" for promoting their implementation, maintaining their relevance, and developing ways to ensure their dissemination to the field. The Evaluator Standards come alive in this book and continue through the work of the Evaluator Competency Think Tank. The focus of this think tank now turns toward the goals of promoting the implementation of these Evaluator Standards and maintaining their currency. Through the evaluator think tank, the board also commits to monitoring the profession to ensure that the identified standards meet the requirements of the profession across time and place. These standards are formally reviewed every three years.

It is the board's intent that these standards defining the knowledge and skills of those who evaluate internal organizational programs, processes, and products serve a variety of settings, users, and uses. It is expected that for-profit and not-for-profit organizations, military, and government agencies evaluating their own internal programs will use these competencies to manage, develop, and implement evaluations. The standards are written for use by novices, experienced or practicing evaluators, managers, academics, consultants, and associations. The uses of these competencies by this constituency are many. For example, the competencies can be used as a basis for developing job requirements, position descriptions, or to direct and manage the work of evaluators. They can serve as benchmarks for self-assessment of one's evaluation skills. These competencies can also serve as the basis for curricula development, curriculum evaluation, student assessment, and research. The utility of this book lies in its clear description of each of the competencies and performance statements so that they can be easily implemented.

To serve the profession, it is the directors' intent to support and mentor organizations and individuals to foster the implementation of these Evaluator Standards. Our directors are advocates for excellence in evaluation performance and are involved in continuous research and publishing, speaking engagements, seminars, workshops, public debate, and using the competencies in their own projects as best practice models.

For current information regarding the organization and its projects, directors, and research, please visit our web site at http://ibstpi.org.

Barbara L. Grabowski
President, ibstpi

Directors of the International Board of Standards for Training, Performance, and Instruction

The board that endorsed and supported the efforts of the subcommittee to develop and validate evaluator competencies and performance standards represented seven countries within corporate, consulting firms, and university settings. This board was also supported by two board advisors and nine ibstpi fellows.

When ibstpi approved (on June 26, 2006) the Evaluator Competencies described in this book, the directors consisted of the following individuals:

Name	Affiliation	Country
Michael F. Beaudoin	University of New England in Portland, Maine	United States
Marcie J. Bober	San Diego State University	United States
Ileana de la Teja	LICEF, Télé-université	Canada
Barbara L. Grabowski	Pennsylvania State University	United States
Bonney Hettinger	Corning, Incorporated	United States
James D. Klein	Arizona State University	United States
Tiffany A. Koszalka	Syracuse University	United States
John O'Connor	O'Connor Consulting, Ltd	United Kingdom
Robert A. Reiser	Florida State University	United States
Darlene F. Russ-Eft	Oregon State University	United States
Roderick Sims	Deakin University	Australia
K R V Subramanian	Ascendum Systems Private Limited	India
Katsuaki Suzuki	Kumamoto University	Japan
Jan Visser	Learning Development Institute	France/USA
Robin Yap	Phronetic International	Canada

There were nine ibstpi fellows, three of whom (Foxon, Spannaus, and Spector, noted by the asterisk) also served as advisor when these competencies were approved:

Dennis Fields	St. Cloud State University	United States
Rob Foshay	Texas Instruments	United States
Marguerite Foxon*	Motorola University	United States
Judith Hale	Hale Associates	United States
Rita Richey	Wayne State University	United States
Dennis Sheriff	Pfizer	United States
Timothy Spannaus*	Institute for Learning and Performance Improvement	United States
J. Michael Spector*	Florida State University	United States
J P Ventosa	Epise	Spain

ACKNOWLEDGMENTS

When the ibstpi Board embarks on a new set of standards, it falls to a small team of board members to commit the next two or three years of their life to working on this project in their "spare" time. No matter how expert in the field they are, they cannot do this work alone, and there is always a large cadre of practitioners and academics who step in behind the team to support, encourage, and contribute from their expertise. Foremost among this group are the members of the expert advisory group who were chosen to represent both the practitioner base and the academic world. We endeavored also to include experts representing regions other than the United States. The team is extremely grateful to the following members of the expert advisory group, whose expertise and patient reviews of our work was critical to its success:

Matt Barney, Sutter Health, United States

Cony Bauer, ImpactResearch, Denmark

Rob Brinkerhoff, Western Michigan University, United States

Jeff Flesher, Underwriters Laboratories, United States

Karin Lundgren, Télé-université, Canada

Jennifer Martineau, Center for Creative Leadership, United States

Hallie Preskill, Claremont Graduate University, United States

Catherine Sleezer, CentriLift Baker-Hughes, United States

Zita Unger, Evaluation Solutions, Australia

Cynthia Weston, McGill University, Canada

Several people helped the team with the global validation. A big Thank You! to Ileana de la Teja (Canada) for translating the competencies into French and to Juan Pablo Ventosa (Spain) and his staff at Epise for the Spanish translation. Also, thanks to Claire Banville (Canada) and Jorge Franchi (United States) for translation reviews. We owe a deep debt of gratitude to Chan Min Kim, Florida State University, who spent hours untangling software glitches and helping us get the survey deployed globally. Finally, Mariah Kraner from Oregon State University and Kristi Andes and Kathy Maher from the American Institutes for Research made sense of the numbers with their data analysis skills. Thank you all!

Each member of the ibstpi Board actively participated in the process. Current and former board members who contributed during the various stages of the project include Michael Beaudoin (United States), Barbara Grabowski (United States), Bonney Hettinger (United States), Jim Klein (United States), Steve Kozlowski (United States), Mark Lee (Australia), John O'Connor (England), Robert Reiser (United States), Rod Sims (Australia), Barbara Sorensen (United States), Tim Spannaus (United States), Michael Spector (United States), Raja Subramanian (India), Jan Visser (France), and Robin Yap (Canada).

Finally, thanks to the many people around the world who reviewed the competencies, provided input and suggestions, and continued to affirm that this was a worthy project. We want to include in these thanks the four anonymous reviewers who gave us some important feedback.

Evaluation Standards Team

Darlene F. Russ-Eft, Ph.D.

Marcie J. Bober, Ph.D.

Ileana de la Teja, Ph.D.

Marguerite Foxon, Ph.D.

Tiffany A. Koszalka, Ph.D.

THE AUTHORS

DARLENE F. RUSS-EFT, PH.D., is associate professor in the Department of Adult Education and Higher Education Leadership in the College of Education at Oregon State University, Corvallis. Her teaching focuses on program evaluation, research methods, and learning theory. Before joining the faculty at Oregon State University, she was division director of research services at AchieveGlobal, the world's largest provider of performance skills training and consulting (focused on leadership, sales, and customer service training).

Dr. Russ-Eft received the 1996 Editor of the Year Award from Times Mirror for her research work and was named Scholar of the Year of the Academy of Human Resource Development (AHRD). She received the American Society for Training and Development (ASTD) Research Article Award for a journal article published in 2004. She holds doctoral and master's degrees from the Department of Psychology at the University of Michigan, Ann Arbor, and a bachelor's degree, with honors, from the Department of Psychology at the College of Wooster, Wooster, Ohio.

An active member of numerous professional organizations, she is the author or coauthor of many articles and essays about research issues, which have appeared in major journals. Her book publications include *A Practical Guide to Needs Assessment* (with K. Gupta and C. M. Sleezer, 2007, Pfeiffer); *Building Evaluation Capacity: 72 Activities for Teaching and Training* (with H. Preskill, 2005, Sage); *Human Resource Development Review* (with H. Preskill and C. Sleezer, 1997, Sage); *What Works: Assessment, Development, and Measurement* (edited with L. J. Bassi, 1997, ASTD); *What Works: Training and Development Practices* (edited with L. J. Bassi, 1997, ASTD); and *Everyone a Leader: A Grassroots Model for the New Workplace* (with H. Bergmann and K. Hurson, 1999, Wiley). She is a speaker at regional, national, and international evaluation, psychology, and training association meetings.

Dr. Russ-Eft is currently a board member and vice president of research for the Academy of Human Resource Development; a current director and board member of the International Board of Standards for Training, Performance, and Instruction (ibstpi); and a current member of the Longitudinal Emergency Medical Technician (EMT) Attributes and Demographics Study committee for the National Registry of EMTs and the National Highway Traffic Safety Administration. She is a member of the review panel for the following journals: *American Journal of Evaluation, International Journal of Training and Development,* and *Human Resource Development International.* She is the immediate past editor of the *Human Resource Development Quarterly,* past chair of the Research Advisory Committee of ASTD, past member of the Research Committee of the Instructional Systems Association, and past member of the board of the American Evaluation Association (AEA).

MARCIE J. BOBER, PH.D., is professor and chair of the Department of Educational Technology at San Diego State University. There she teaches field-based courses where students work directly with community-based clients (SeaWorld, San Diego City Schools, Kyocera Wireless, International Rescue Center) to conduct both voluntary and mandated evaluation studies. Dr. Bober is a frequent contributor to professional journals and books; her most recent publications have focused on team-based activities to promote engaged learning, ensuring quality in technology-focused professional development, and the complexities of measuring technological literacy.

Since 1995, Dr. Bober has served as lead evaluator on several federal grants targeting our public schools—for the most part, initiatives to stimulate effective use of advanced technologies in the classroom and positively affect student learning and workforce readiness. She is also a frequent presenter at technology conferences focused on the design, development, and evaluation of technologies aimed at improved human performance and consults extensively with organizations interested in assessing technology's impact on productivity and efficiency, creativity and risk taking, morale, and group interactions.

In addition to her work as an ibstpi Board member, Dr. Bober is cochair of the AEA's Integrating Technology into Evaluation topical interest group. She also is active in the Association for Educational Communications and Technology (AECT) and the American Association of School Administrators (where she served for several years on its Technology Advisory Committee).

Dr. Bober received her doctorate in learning and instructional technology from Arizona State University, Tempe, and her master's in educational technology from San Diego State University. She has served as a faculty fellow for three different agencies or groups at San Diego

State: the June Burnett Institute for Children, Youth, and Families; the Center for Teacher and Learning; and the Education Center on Computational Science and Engineering. Each affiliation was evaluation focused, resulting in strategies to improve instructional assessment, program processes and client communications, and peer feedback systems.

ILEANA DE LA TEJA, PH.D., is associate professor and researcher at Télé-université, the distance university of the University of Quebec in Montreal. She received her master's degree and doctorate in educational technology at the University of Montreal. Her research interests include the evaluation of virtual learning environments, evaluation of competencies, competency modeling, and the design of tools and methods for online instructional designers. Her research work has resulted in numerous publications, including the award-winning *Instructor Competencies* book (coauthored with J. Klein, M. Spector, and B. Grabowski, 2004, Information Age). She has also coedited a special issue of *Education and Program Planning* that focused on the evaluation of learning technology.

Dr. de la Teja has been a director of ibstpi since 2000 and served as secretary from 2001 to 2005. She has also participated in the evaluation of the certification tests of the Barreau du Quebec and in the elaboration of competency models for various professional associations. She has coordinated a Canadian-based effort in two projects aiming to adapt and implement methods and technology, using a competency-based approach, to a network of universities in Chile (REUNA). Among her latest projects is the design of instructional scenarios based on the IMS-Learning Design standards.

Other professional activities include participation in the *Educational, Technology, Research, and Development* (ETR&D) journal board and being a consultant to the International Institute of Telecommunications for the evaluation of competencies in corporate settings.

Dr. de la Teja received a license degree in communication and journalism (1980) and worked for years as an announcer-producer at the Canadian Broadcasting Corporation for Radio Canada International.

MARGUERITE FOXON, PH.D., is a highly respected evaluation and performance improvement specialist who brings 25 years of experience in managing large-scale evaluation and global leadership development programs in Australia and the United States. She received her doctorate from Florida State University, Tallahassee, in instructional systems, specializing in research on transfer evaluation and action planning. In 2006 she received the Outstanding Alumnus award. She has three graduate degrees from Australia and New Zealand and has been active in many professional associations during her career.

Dr. Foxon has lived and worked in three countries, delivered conference presentations in nine, and authored or coauthored more than a dozen articles, three book chapters, and two books: *Instructional Design Competencies: The Standards,* third edition (with R. C. Richey and D. C. Fields, 2001, ERIC Clearinghouse on Information and Technology) and *Training Manager Competencies: The Standards,* second edition (with R. C. Richey, R. C. Roberts, and T. Spannaus, 2003, ERIC Clearinghouse on Information and Technology). Dr. Foxon was an ibstpi director for nine years and has been elected as an ibstpi fellow for life. She is listed in the *International Who's Who of Professionals* and in *Who's Who Among Executive and Professional Women.*

In the United States, Dr. Foxon worked at Motorola for 13 years and most recently was manager of Global Leadership Content and Evaluation. Before that, she worked with PriceWaterhouseCoopers in Australia, where she was national director of education. She is now consulting in evaluation and needs assessment through her own company, Performance Improvement Consulting.

TIFFANY A. KOSZALKA, PH.D., is associate professor of instructional design, development, and evaluation at Syracuse University. She has worked in instructional design and technology integration for more than 20 years. She earned a doctorate from Pennsylvania State University, University Park, in instructional systems with a minor in cultural anthropology. Dr. Koszalka has managed and evaluated large-scale training projects that integrated leading-edge technologies into instructional solutions for several organizations, including Andersen Consulting, Pepsi-Cola, Mobil, and Johnson & Johnson Diagnostics. During the past several years, she shifted her attention to K–12 and higher education environments. Dr. Koszalka's research agenda is studying and evaluating the integration of technology resources into instructional and learning environments, specifically investigating learning in complex domains. She often serves in assessment and research roles and consults on instructional design, technology integration, and human performance efforts. She is currently the ibspti treasurer.

INTRODUCTION

Various books currently exist that focus on the processes associated with evaluation. But few books outline the competencies needed by evaluators to undertake evaluations. Furthermore, nothing exists to describe the competencies needed by evaluators who work within organizational settings. Having such a book would enable individuals and organizations to identify those with the competencies and skills to undertake needed evaluations. Furthermore, universities offering evaluation programs and courses can use these competencies to aid in program development, as part of the curriculum for their courses, and as an assessment tool to identify student progress toward competency development.

Recognizing the above-described need, the International Board of Standards for Training, Performance, and Instruction (ibstpi®; see http://ibstpi.org) launched a project in June 2004 to identify the competencies needed by those undertaking evaluation efforts. In some instances, these may be internal evaluators or staff within the organization. In other cases, these may be external evaluators or consultants from outside the organization who are asked to undertake the evaluation. In both cases, though, such evaluations focus on programs, processes, and products within the organization and can include the following settings:

- For-profit and not-for-profit organizations
- The military
- Government agencies evaluating their own internal programs

The competencies needed by such individuals are different from those needed by evaluators examining the effectiveness of large-scale statewide or national programs often funded by government departments or agencies. Competencies for such large-scale evaluations are provided by the American Evaluation Association, for example, and are covered in numerous textbooks on program evaluation.

Selected members of the ibstpi Board drafted the competencies. These were reviewed by selected evaluation experts and revised. The revised competencies were distributed in English, French, and Spanish, and evaluators throughout the world responded by indicating the importance of each of the statements. These validated competencies form the basis for the book.

Several academic programs in the United States and abroad have aligned their programs with other ibstpi competencies (e.g., training, managing, and instructional design). We expect that this will happen for these competencies as well.

PURPOSE OF THE BOOK

In this book, we present the validated Evaluator Competencies and describe each of these competencies. We also discuss the challenges and obstacles in conducting such evaluations within dynamic, changing organizations. Furthermore, we identify alternative approaches to overcoming these challenges and obstacles. Our goals for the book are

- To inform current and future human resource development (HRD), human performance technologists (HPT), and human resource management (HRM) professionals about the competencies needed to undertake evaluations within organizations

- To provide information about and strategies for achieving these competencies

- To serve as a text for practitioners and for graduate-level courses in evaluation, including those associated with HRD, HPT, and HRM programs

- To serve as the basis for HRD, HPT, and HRM curriculum development

SUMMARY OF THE BOOK

In Part I of the book, we discuss the development, validation, and application of the ibstpi Evaluator Competencies. The first chapter begins by providing an overview to the practice of evaluation within organizational settings. Various approaches and theories of evaluation are reviewed. In the second chapter, we introduce the need for an examination of competencies among evaluators. We examine various sources to help identify these competencies. The third chapter contains a brief summary of the ibstpi approach to competency identification and validation.

At the end of that chapter is a list of the ibstpi Evaluator Competencies, along with the performance statements. In the fourth chapter, we discuss each of the domains, competencies, and performance statements and provide suggestions to improve practice. Ways in which the ibstpi Evaluator Competencies can be used are described in Chapter 5.

In Part II, we present the details of the validation effort, beginning with (in Chapter 6) a description of some of the foundational research supporting and contributing to the development process. In Chapter 7, we present the details of the validation study, and in the final chapter (Chapter 8), we discuss the future of evaluation and the evaluator competencies.

In the appendixes are provided helpful tools and resources for evaluators: a history and description of ibstpi (Appendix A), a glossary of terms used in this book (Appendix B), a discussion of the separate survey undertaken on various evaluation tools and approaches (Appendix C), an annotated bibliography of resources linked to the evaluator competencies and performance statements (Appendix D), and a list of professional associations relevant for evaluators working within organizational settings (Appendix E).

READING THE BOOK

The book can be read cover to cover for those who are interested in all of the details. Those who are mostly concerned about the competencies and their application should focus on Chapters 4 and 5. Chapters 1, 2, and 3 may also prove helpful for application and understanding, and Appendix D may provide useful resources for further understanding about evaluation and evaluator competencies. Those who are interested in the details of the validation effort should turn to Chapters 3, 6, and 7. Those who are interested in ibstpi and its approach to evaluation may want to examine Chapters 2 and 7 as well as Appendix A.

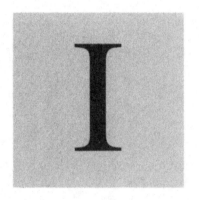

THE IBSTPI®
EVALUATOR
COMPETENCIES:
DEVELOPMENT,
INTERPRETATION,
AND APPLICATION

CHAPTER

THE PRACTICE OF EVALUATION IN ORGANIZATIONS

This chapter will enable you to accomplish the following:

- Identify several major evaluation approaches used within organizational settings
- Describe some similarities among the approaches
- Describe some differences among the approaches

Various professionals and managers within organizations are increasingly called on to undertake evaluations of organizational programs and processes. This emphasis comes from a variety of sources. In some cases, it arises because of pressure from executives. For example, a study by the Conference Board (Gates, 2005) found that executives plan to make increasing use of human capital metrics. The explanation for this interest by executives involves the role that such measures and evaluation play in helping the organization achieve its strategic goals. In other cases, line managers, including those in human resources (HR), human resource development (HRD), and human performance technology (HPT), recognize the importance of measuring the effects and impacts of their interventions. Such information can be used to determine what changes, if any, are needed in the interventions to meet their objectives. Thus, knowledge and skills in evaluation appear to be of increasing importance within organizations.

Given the importance of evaluations done within organizational contexts, this book provides some background on such work. More important, this book presents and discusses competencies needed by those undertaking evaluations within organizational settings, whether these are for-profit, nonprofit, governmental, or military organizations. Such evaluators are, however, focused on examining internal organizational programs, processes, and products. Thus, the competencies described in this book are not necessarily relevant to evaluators who are examining local, state, or national programs. So as an example, the national-level Department of Education may provide funding for programs aimed at reducing adult illiteracy, and there may be an evaluation being undertaken of that program. The competencies and standards that the evaluator should use for such an evaluation are typically described by some national evaluation association, such as the American Evaluation Association, the Australasian Evaluation Society, the Canadian Evaluation Society, and so forth. At the same time, however, that same Department of Education may provide internal staff training on conflict management and may ask a staff person or an external consultant to evaluate it. The competencies described in this book are relevant and applicable to such an evaluator. Furthermore, it should be recognized that although the example describes a governmental organization, such internally focused evaluations take place in a variety of organizations that may be small or large and that may provide products or services locally, nationally, or globally.

The purpose of this chapter is to provide a brief overview of the theory and research that exists concerning evaluations within organizations. It should be recognized that evaluation work focused within organizational settings has tended to follow a different evolution and history than that characterized by program evaluation. Russ-Eft and Preskill (2001) provided a comprehensive examination of the development of the field of evaluation and of the specialized area focused on evaluations within organizational settings. This chapter does not replicate the description of that history, but instead provides a brief overview focused on evaluations within organizations. Furthermore, it presents this overview following the recent suggestion by Wang and Spitzer (2005) that the field can be characterized by three types of approaches: (a) "practice-oriented atheoretical," (b) "process-driven operational," and (c) "research-oriented, practice-based comprehensive" (p. 6).

PRACTICE-ORIENTED ATHEORETICAL APPROACHES

Much of the work on evaluation within organizational settings began with Donald Kirkpatrick, who focused on whether programs are achieving their objectives. He created a taxonomy that he called a "four-step approach" to evaluation and has more recently called "levels of evaluation" or the "four-level model." His work was initially published in a series of articles in 1959 and 1960, and it was updated in 1994. Some other practice-oriented approaches, many of them variants of the Kirkpatrick approach, will also be mentioned.

Kirkpatrick's Four-Level Evaluation Model

Kirkpatrick (1959a, b; 1960a, b) described the outcomes of training as focused on *reactions, learning, behavior,* and *results,* and he proposed that evaluations of such training should measure each of these outcomes. A level 1 evaluation gathers reactions to the training, a level 2 evaluation determines trainees' learning, a level 3 evaluation measures the behavior of trainees (typically on the job), and a level 4 evaluation examines the business results from training.

Kirkpatrick's taxonomy has had extensive application in training evaluations, and this primarily stems from the fact that it is easy to understand. In 1993, Kraiger, Ford, and Salas asserted that "Kirkpatrick's recommendations continue to represent the state-of-the art training evaluation" (p. 311); however, they did suggest some improvements in the taxonomy. Later, Hilbert, Preskill, and Russ-Eft (1997) reviewed 57 journal articles in the training, performance, and psychology literatures that discussed or mentioned training evaluation models. Of those, 44 (or 77 percent) included Kirkpatrick's model (either alone or in comparison with another model). A mere 13 articles discussed a model other than Kirkpatrick's.

Although Kirkpatrick's approach has been discussed in the literature, organizations have not tended to implement all four levels. Training interventions, in particular, are typically evaluated at the reaction and learning levels, with only some attention paid to the behavioral outcomes. For example, Taylor, Russ-Eft, and Chan (2005) undertook a meta-analysis of studies, both published and unpublished, that evaluated the effectiveness of behavior-modeling training. Of these studies, 52 measured attitudes, 14 measured declarative knowledge, 32 measured procedural knowledge, 66 measured job behavior, and none measured business results. The reliance on reaction and learning measures may be due to the perceived difficulty and cost in measuring performance or behavior and organizational benefits. Some would consider such a result to be ironic because they would view improvements to the business as representing the business case for a learning or training investment.

Kirkpatrick's approach to evaluation has served as the basis for the development of other similar models for use in corporate, military, or small organizational settings. The remainder of this section describes some of these models, approaches, and taxonomies.

Navy Civilian Personnel Command Model

Similar to the Kirkpatrick approach, the Navy Civilian Personnel Command model examines knowledge and competencies gained during training (Erickson, 1990), but the measurement of those knowledge and competencies involves intensive testing. In this particular evaluation, trainees in staffing and placement experience intensive interviews three to six months after training. The interviews present real-life situations, and trainees must explain how to handle those situations to a subject-matter expert. Such an approach more closely approximates the transfer situation than does a paper-and-pencil test.

Training Effectiveness Evaluation System

The Training Effectiveness Evaluation System (Swanson & Sleezer, 1987) recommends measuring participants' and supervisors' satisfaction; trainees' knowledge and skills; and organizational, process, job, and financial performance. Four separate tools, then, are suggested: two satisfaction measures (participant and supervisor), a trainee learning measure, and a financial performance measure. Scores from each of the tools are then assessed before and after an intervention.

Hamblin's Five-Level Model

Hamblin (1974) proposed a five-level model similar to Kirkpatrick's, suggesting that evaluations measure reactions, learning, job behavior, and organizational impact (noneconomic outcomes of training). In addition, however, he indicated that there should be a level 5; this level should measure "ultimate value variables" or "human good" (economic outcomes).

Kaufman, Keller, Watkins Five-Level Model

Kaufman and Keller (1994) and Kaufman, Keller, and Watkins (1995) proposed a model that expanded on the ideas of both Kirkpatrick and Hamblin. They suggested the levels of Enabling and Reaction, Acquisition, Application, and Organizational Outputs—again, conceptually similar to Kirkpatrick. In addition, they recognized the societal impact and included Societal Outcomes as a fifth level. By adding it, they take into account the societal impact of training or of any HRD intervention. Such a model recognizes that organizations and the programs and processes within those organizations can affect clients and the larger society. According to Kaufman, Keller, and Watkins (1995), such Societal Outcomes or "megalevel" (p. 375) provides evidence of the ways in which the organization benefits the society.

Swanson and Holton's Results Model

Swanson and Holton (1999, p. 8) claimed that "assessment and evaluation are different. Assessment of results is a core organizational process. Evaluation is optional." They then proceeded to describe approaches to measuring performance results in terms of systems outcomes and financial outcomes, learning results in terms of knowledge and expertise outcomes, and reaction results in terms of participant and stakeholder outcomes. They also detailed specific measurement approaches such as the critical outcome technique, auditing program practices and effectiveness, certification of core expertise, and assessing performance drivers.

PROCESS-DRIVEN OPERATIONAL APPROACHES

The Wang and Spitzer (2005) conceptualization of process-driven operational approaches tends to limit examination to issues related to return on investment (ROI). By taking a broader view, however, we can identify various other approaches that focus on processes, either within programs or within the evaluation.

Brinkerhoff's Stage Model

Brinkerhoff (1988, 1989) suggested a cyclical approach in which every phase of a program can be evaluated. His six-stage model begins with goal setting or needs analysis. In this stage, the evaluation involves identifying the training needs before designing a program. In the next stage, the evaluation examines the program's design. The third stage evaluates the training program's operation or implementation, and the later stages may be considered similar to the outcomes in Kirkpatrick's approach. This stage model provides a type of formative evaluation in that the results can be used to aid in decision making and improvement through the design and implementation of the program.

Input, Process, Output Model

Bushnell (1990) described the Input, Process, Output Model as IBM's corporate education strategy for the year 2000 and, similar to Brinkerhoff's stage model, views the evaluation as a cyclical process. This model also appears related to the context, input, process, and product (or CIPP) evaluation suggested by Stufflebeam (1983, 2000). The Input, Process, Output model begins by examining the input factors that may affect a program's effectiveness, such as trainee qualifications, program design, instructor quality and qualifications, materials quality, facilities, and equipment. The process factors are then examined, and these include such variables as the planning, developing, and delivery of the training. The results can then be evaluated and divided or organized into the outputs and the outcomes. Outputs are considered the short-term results and include trainee reactions, knowledge and skill gains, and job performance improvement; outcomes, or long-term results, include what might be considered business results, such as profits, customer satisfaction, and productivity.

Stages of Transfer Model

Foxon's (1994) Stages of Transfer Model focuses on the transfer resulting from a training intervention, and it views transfer as a process rather than an outcome. The stages of transfer move from conscious intention to unconscious maintenance, with each stage affected by supporting or inhibiting factors.

> Stage 1: Intention to transfer begins with the decision and the motivation to apply newly acquired knowledge and skills. The training environment, work environment, and organizational environment support or inhibit this intention.

> Stage 2: Initiation occurs with the first attempt to apply new knowledge and skills at the job. The organizational climate, trainee characteristics, training design, and training delivery can support or inhibit this initiation.

Stage 3: Partial transfer takes place when some of the knowledge and skills are learned or are applied inconsistently. Skill mastery, the opportunity and motivation to utilize the learning, and the confidence to apply skills and knowledge support or inhibit this partial transfer.

Stage 4: Conscious maintenance occurs with the conscious application of what was learned in training, and this is supported or inhibited by the trainee's motivation and skills.

Stage 5: Unconscious maintenance occurs when the new knowledge and skill are integrated into the work routine.

Return on Investment

Literature describing the evaluation of business results, financial results, and ROI has become increasingly popular. Phillips and Phillips (2005, 2006) have written extensively about ROI and consider this to equate to Kirkpatrick's level 5 evaluation. At this level, "impact measures are converted to monetary values and compared with the fully loaded program costs" (Phillips & Phillips, 2006, p. 3). Evaluation at this level is typically represented by the benefit-cost ratio (BCR) or by ROI. The following provides the basic formula:

$$\text{BCR} = \text{Program Benefits}/\text{Program Costs}$$

$$\text{ROI} = [\text{Program Benefits}/\text{Program Costs}] \times 100$$

Despite the interest in ROI and cost-benefit kinds of outcomes, well-designed and well-documented ROI evaluation efforts are hard to find, particularly in relation to programs in which outcomes are focused on attitudes rather than knowledge or skill. It can even be difficult to measure the ROI of leadership development programs, which is where many executives are concerned about evaluation. Bartel (1997), however, identified some key attributes for determining ROI, specifically of training interventions. One key recommendation is that evaluators interested in financial benefits or ROI use the net present value or the internal rate-of-return method when determining the ROI of training. Both of these methods take into account the time value of money.

RESEARCH-ORIENTED, PRACTICE-BASED COMPREHENSIVE APPROACHES

Wang and Spitzer (2005) suggest that some of the more recent approaches tend to have a practice base but are also research and theory driven. A more appropriate characterization, however, might be that they are focused on systemic issues within the organizational setting. In this section, we review some of those approaches.

Systemic Model of Factors Predicting Employee Training Outcomes

Richey (1992) described a Systemic Model of Factors Predicting Employee Training Outcomes. The model focuses on factors affecting training outcomes, particularly the trainee characteristics and perceptions of the organization. Thus, it posits that the trainee attitudes are affected by such background characteristics as age, education, previous training, ability to learn, and motivation. Furthermore, these attitudes are also affected by the working conditions and management approach. Although instructional design and delivery may affect training outcomes, it is these trainee attitudes that have a direct effect on knowledge and behavior resulting from training.

Learning Outcomes Model

Kraiger, Ford, and Salas (1993) suggested that training evaluations should focus on the learning outcomes. Furthermore, they argued that training evaluation lacked theoretically based models. They used cognitive, social, and instructional psychology and human factors to determine the relevant outcomes. These were identified as cognitive, skill-based, and affective learning outcomes, and potential measures were suggested for each.

Training Efficiency and Effectiveness Model

Lincoln and Dunet (1995) recommended that evaluation should take place throughout the training process, with results continuously informing next steps. Their model consists of evaluation stages as analysis, development, delivery, and results. The approach suggests that the evaluator identify all stakeholders in the program and the evaluation. These views and information needs of these stakeholders need to be considered in the design, development, and implementation of the evaluation.

Brinkerhoff's Impact Map

Brinkerhoff and Gill (1994) suggested that too often the wrong people get sent to the training or that the right people attend but there are factors preventing their use of the training, such as poor program design, inadequate instructors, the lack of supervisory or peer support, a fear of failure, or a system that punishes the new behaviors. In such cases, the intervention can have little or no impact. As a result, Brinkerhoff and Gill introduced the notion of an *impact map*, which can be viewed as similar to the idea of evaluability assessment introduced by Joseph Wholey (1975, 1976, 1979). In this case, the evaluator creates a "map" showing the entire process from an input phase to the desired outcomes. This map can then help to identify both the process and the factors that can affect the outcomes.

Brinkerhoff's Success Case Evaluation Method

More recently, Brinkerhoff (2003, 2006) introduced what he calls "the success case method." This method enables the evaluator to examine the ways in which the training is or is not aligned with the business strategy. It begins by recognizing that "programs are almost never completely successful such that 100% of the participants use learning on the job in a way that drives business results. Similarly, almost no program is ever a 100% failure such that no trainee ever uses anything for any worthwhile outcome" (Brinkerhoff, 2005, p. 92). Rather than gather superficial information regarding all trainees, the method involves examining the successful and the unsuccessful cases. This information can then be used to document the individual and business effects and can identify the factors that support or hinder those effects. It also provides impact data demonstrating the measurable impact of the intervention on the organization.

Holton's HRD Evaluation Research and Measurement Model

Holton's model (1996) argued that the Kirkpatrick model is really a taxonomy. As a more comprehensive model, he proposed that the three outcomes of training (learning, individual performance, and organizational results) are influenced by primary and secondary factors. More recently, Holton (2005) has elaborated on the original model. Although the outcomes remain as learning, individual performance, and organizational performance, the various factors influencing these involve ability, environment, motivation, and secondary influences on each of these outcomes.

Preskill and Russ-Eft Systems Model

Preskill and Russ-Eft (2003, 2005) and Russ-Eft and Preskill (2001, 2005) recommended that evaluations within organizations use a systems model. Such a model recognizes not only the various factors affecting the individuals and the program or process but also the factors that influence the evaluation itself. Thus, the knowledge and competence of the evaluator and the procedures used in the evaluation can affect the outcomes and the findings as much as the design of the program, the motivation of the participants, and the support from peers and supervisors. In addition, the context affecting the organization, such as the competitive environment and the views of customers, may also affect the evaluation and its outcomes. Finally, such a systems model recognizes that these factors both influence the evaluation and the outcomes and are influenced by the evaluation and its outcomes.

CONCLUSIONS

A variety of approaches to evaluation exist for use by evaluators working within many different organizational settings, including small, medium, and large companies; local, state, and national government agencies; and local, regional, national, and international nongovernmental organizations. As more and more of these organizations undertake evaluation efforts, the various approaches to evaluation continue to evolve. Furthermore, this evolution now suggests that organizations and the programs within them are complex systems that are difficult both to examine and to evaluate. Thus, there is a need to determine the competencies required by those who undertake evaluations within such contexts.

QUESTIONS FOR CONSIDERATION

What are two different evaluation approaches that you might use, and on what basis would you make a choice?

Choose two of the evaluation approaches that you could use in your organization and identify the benefits and drawbacks of each approach.

Describe how you would combine two or more of these approaches for use in an organization.

CHAPTER

2

IN SEARCH OF EVALUATOR COMPETENCIES

This chapter will enable you to accomplish the following:

- Identify evaluator competencies grounded in ethical codes of conduct
- Identify evaluator competencies derived from evaluation textbooks
- Identify evaluator competencies derived from academic and certificate programs
- Compare and contrast competencies from various sources

Because we are focused on determining evaluator competencies, we might simply pose the question: What are the knowledge, skills, and attitudes (or competencies) needed to undertake such evaluation? To answer this question, it would seem appropriate to turn to the literature on evaluation. Worthen and Sanders (1991) described some evidence of professionalization of evaluation: career opportunities, preparation programs, university-based programs, methodological developments, and most important, the adoption of *The Standards for Evaluations of Educational Programs, Projects, and Materials* (Joint Committee, 1981;

and later the *Program Evaluation Standards*). Nevertheless, King, Stevahn, Ghere, and Minnema (2001, p. 230) stated that "the standards do not directly address the competencies an evaluator needs to function effectively in specific contexts." In particular, *The Program Evaluation Standards* (Joint Committee on Standards for Educational Evaluation, 1994) and the *Guiding Principles for Evaluators* (American Evaluation Association, 2004) tend to address issues related to evaluations of large-scale federal- and state-funded programs.

In the present chapter, we describe the process of determining the competencies needed to undertake evaluation within the organizational settings—that is, the competencies that form the basis for this book. Such settings include for-profit organizations, not-for-profit organizations, government, and military agencies (examining their own internal programs, processes, and products). These are in contrast to large-scale evaluations of government programs that tend to be the focus of much of the program evaluation literature. We examine three streams of literature to attempt to answer this question: (1) the standards for evaluators developed by various national and international professional associations, (2) frameworks proposed for evaluator tasks and skills as outlined in various evaluation texts, and (3) content for various certification programs in evaluation. Furthermore, we examine each of these streams through the initial competency work by King et al. (2001) and through the initial efforts by the International Board of Standards for Training, Performance, and Instruction (ibstpi®). We conclude with some recommendations for an empirical data-gathering effort to clarify and validate these evaluator competencies. This chapter is based on a paper titled "In Search of Evaluator Competencies" presented at the Sixth Annual Conference of Human Resource Development Across Europe, held at the University of Leeds, Leeds, United Kingdom, May 2005.

NEED TO DETERMINE EVALUATOR COMPETENCIES

Because ibstpi's concern is with issues related to training, performance, and instruction, the organization focused its initial competency development efforts specifically on those issues. Thus, ibstpi developed and more recently revised competencies for Instructional Designers (Richey, Fields, & Foxon, 2001), Training Managers (Foxon, Richey, Roberts, & Spannaus, 2003), and Instructors (Klein, Spector, Grabowski, & de la Teja, 2004). In the course of working on revisions of the various competencies, ibstpi realized that evaluation had come to play a more important role in each of these fields. Initially, ibstpi examined the fields of human resource development (HRD) and evaluation to determine whether competencies and standards existed that would be relevant to those engaged in evaluations related to training, performance, and instruction.

The separate fields of HRD and of evaluation have been developing and becoming increasingly professional, yet each lacked a clear competency model for evaluation within organizational settings. Burns, Russ-Eft, and Wright (2001), Ruona and Rusaw (2001), and Russ-Eft (2004c) identified some of the characteristics of a profession; two of these characteristics involve an organized and specialized body of knowledge and a defined area of competence. Ruona and Rusaw (2001) further identified specific steps taken to address each of the characteristics. Thus, they suggested that evidence for the first characteristic (that of an organized and specialized body of knowledge) appeared with the creation of a new professional association along with regional conferences and various journals. As for evidence of an area of competence, they suggested the competency models of McLagan (1989) and Rothwell (1996). It should be noted that although these models include evaluation, this particular competency area is not fully described.

As for the field of evaluation, Worthen and Sanders (1991) provided arguments to support evaluation as a separate profession. Nevertheless, King et al. (2001, p. 230) indicated that "one noticeable deficiency is a coherent and widely accepted set of the unique skills and knowledge that distinguishes professional evaluators." In considering the issue of certifying evaluators, Smith (1999) suggested some approaches to identifying such evaluator competencies. One approach might be to use the AEA *Guiding Principles*; however, she discounted this particular listing as too general to be of use. A second approach would be to ask evaluators to generate such a listing, but this may be limited by those who respond. A third approach would be to undertake some sort of job analyses that evaluation users or employers consider critical. Indeed, Russ-Eft (1995, 2004a) provided discussion of these last two types of approach and an example focused on customer service competencies. As another example, the government-sponsored replacement to the *Dictionary of Occupational Titles,* O*Net, has a public domain taxonomy of various job competencies (http://www .onetcenter.org). King et al. (2001) undertook an exploratory study with 31 evaluators in the Minneapolis-St. Paul area to determine whether evaluation professions could reach consensus on a proposed taxonomy of competencies. None of these evaluators worked within a for-profit organization, and only seven participants worked within a government agency.

Both HRD and evaluation are increasingly being recognized as professional fields, and evaluation within organizational settings is of increasing interest and concern to both fields. However, neither of the fields has examined the competencies needed by those who undertake evaluations within organizational settings. It is time to begin to determine the competencies of those who undertake evaluations within organizations, whether these are for-profit or nonprofit organizations or government agencies. Indeed, recognizing this need, ibstpi commissioned the study described in this book to identify and validate such competencies. Thus, this chapter represents an initial step in the larger competency study and validation effort.

RESEARCH QUESTIONS FOR THE EXAMINATION OF THE LITERATURE

The major question guiding this research was, What are the competencies needed by those who undertake evaluations within organizational settings? This particular study aimed at examining available literature to determine whether these sources can aid in this identification. Therefore, a more specific research question for this study was, What competencies for organizational evaluators can be identified through an examination of standards from national and international associations, from evaluation textbooks, and from academic and certificate programs? A second question for this study was, To what extent do the competencies identified from these various sources agree with those identified by King et al. (2001)?

APPROACH TO THE LITERATURE STUDY

We begin this section by defining what is meant by competencies and competency modeling. We then provide the details of the literature search process.

Definitions and Processes for Competency Modeling

McClelland (1973) suggested that competencies provide an unbiased approach to predicting job performance. Klemp (1980, p. 21) defined a competency as "an underlying characteristic of a person which results in effective and/or superior performance on the job." Stephenson and Raven (2001, p. ix) described competencies as "key skills, core skills, enterprise skills, life skills, and personal transferable skills." McLagan (1997) suggested that competencies might be defined in one of six ways: (1) job tasks; (2) work results; (3) outputs; (4) knowledge, skills, and attitudes; (5) qualities of superior performance; and (6) some grouping of attributes.

In contrast, ibstpi (Richey, Fields, & Foxon, 2001, p. 31) defines a competency as "a set of related knowledge, skills, and attitudes that enable an individual to effectively perform the activities of a given occupation or job function to the standards expected in employment."

The ibstpi competency development model described in Richey, Fields, and Foxon (2001) includes three phases. The first phase examines current practices focused on standards of performance, ethics and values, and finally, a vision of the future. The second phase identifies the knowledge, skills, and attitudes that represent competent performance. The third phase then validates the identified skills, knowledge, and attitudes. The literature study represented the first two phases of this development effort to yield a listing of domains of performance and competencies that can undergo worldwide validation at a later date.

Literature Search Process

The study consisted of an examination of available documents from national and international associations, books on evaluation, and academic and certificate programs. Russ-Eft (2004b) provided a base for examining the ethical guidelines and standards adopted by various national evaluation associations, such as the African Evaluation Guidelines, the American Evaluation Association (AEA)'s *Guiding Principles,* the Canadian Evaluation Society's Guidelines for Ethical Conduct, and the German Evaluation Society Standards for Evaluation. In addition, information available on the web site of the AEA was examined. That site identifies the various national evaluation associations. From these listings, further web searches were undertaken to locate any additional statements of standards. The AEA web site also provides a listing of various academic programs with some of the content of those programs. To this listing, some web searches identified other academic and certificate programs. The books were limited to those that were considered basic texts providing general overview on evaluation, with particular emphasis on those that attend to evaluation within organizational settings.

RESULTS OF THE LITERATURE STUDY

The following paragraphs present the results of the literature search. These results are divided into the standards identified from various professional associations, those emerging from various textbooks, and those appearing in various academic and certificate courses. These standards from these sources are then compared with each other and with the one competency study appearing in the literature, that of King et al. (2001). All of this serves as a foundation for the ibstpi Evaluator Competency development and validation.

Standards for Evaluators Developed by Various National and International Associations

Table 2.1 presents the results from the standards for evaluators identified by various professional organizations operating in locations throughout the world. Many similarities appeared among the different statements. For example, all of the standards appeared to address the issue of professional foundations and the basis for professional competence. Indeed, several of these used and adapted statements from similar organizations. Thus, the Deutsche Gesellschaft für Evaluation and the African Evaluation Association both adapted the previously written Program Evaluation Standards (Joint Committee on Standards for Educational Evaluation, 1994). This makes comparison among the various standards somewhat easier to undertake.

These standards appear to provide a useful starting point, but they do not seem to go into some of the content areas needed by evaluators. For example, evaluators must be able to use a variety of quantitative and qualitative methods (Russ-Eft & Preskill, 2001), and yet none of these standards specifically addresses such methods or even data collection or modern measurement approaches. At the same time, some of these standards pointed to issues related to social responsibility. This presumes that all evaluations have a component of "social responsibility," and that may be of little importance or even controversial for evaluators operating within an organization setting. Perhaps this analysis shows that these standards tend to be broad and general in order to cover the many

TABLE 2.1 Comparison of Various Ethical Codes or Standards

Standards Categories / Domains and Competencies	AHRD Standards (1999)	AEA Guiding Principles (2004)	Program Evaluation Standards (1994; modified by DeGEval, 2001; modified by the African Evaluation Association, 2002)	CES Guidelines for Ethical Conduct (n.d.)
Professional Foundations and Competence ■ Communicate accurately and effectively ■ Observe ethical standards ■ Obtain and maintain needed skills	**Competence** ■ Boundaries of competence ■ Maintenance of competence ■ Basis for research and professional judgments ■ Description of HRD professional's work ■ Data collection ■ Responsibility ■ Avoidance of false or deceptive statements	**Systematic Inquiry and Competence** A1: Adhere to technical standards A2: Explore evaluation questions and approaches A3: Communicate methods and approaches accurately and in sufficient detail B1: Possess appropriate education, abilities, skills, and experience B2: Ensure and demonstrate cultural competence B3: Practice within limits of training and competence B4: Maintain and improve competencies	**Utility and Accuracy** U2: Evaluator credibility (and competence) U3: Information scope and selection A1: Program documentation (description of evaluand) A2: Context analysis A3: Described purposes and procedures A4: Defensible information sources (disclosure of information sources) A5: Valid measurement A6: Reliable measurement A7: Systematic control (systematic data review) A8: Analysis of quantitative information A9: Analysis of qualitative information A10: Justified conclusions A12: Metaevaluation	**Competence** ■ Apply systematic methods ■ Possess content knowledge ■ Continuously improve practice

(Continued)

Program Evaluation Standards (1994; modified by DeGEval, 2001; modified by the African Evaluation Association, 2002)

Standards Categories / Domains and Competencies	AHRD Standards (1999)	AEA Guiding Principles (2004)	Program Evaluation Standards (1994; modified by DeGEval, 2001; modified by the African Evaluation Association, 2002)	CES Guidelines for Ethical Conduct (n.d.)
Professional Responsibility, Integrity, Accountability ■ Accurately represent skills ■ Disclose conflicts of interest ■ Negotiate honestly ■ Communicate accurately and fairly	**Integrity and Professional Responsibility** ■ Misuse of HRD professional's work ■ Multiple relationships ■ Consultations and referrals ■ Third party request for services ■ Advertising and other public statements ■ Publication of work	**Integrity / Honesty** C1: Negotiate honestly on costs, tasks, limitations, scope of results, and data use C2: Disclose any conflicts of interest C3: Record changes in project plans and reasons for changes C4: Communicate explicitly on own, client, and stakeholder interests in evaluation conduct and outcomes C5: Avoid misrepresentation and misuse of procedures, data, or findings C6: Communicate concerns about misleading information C7: Disclose sources of financial support for evaluation	**Feasibility, Propriety, and Accuracy** F2: Political viability (diplomatic conduct) F3: Cost effectiveness (evaluation efficiency) P2: Formal agreements P4: Unbiased conduct and reporting P5: Complete and fair assessment (complete and fair investigation) P6: Disclosure of findings P7: Conflict of interest P8: Fiscal responsibility A5: Valid information A10: Justified conclusions A11: Objective reporting A12: Metaevaluation	**Integrity and Accountability** ■ Accurately represent skills and knowledge ■ Declare conflict of interest ■ Confer on contractual decisions ■ Provide information for selection of strategies and methods ■ Be responsible for clear, accurate, and fair presentation ■ Be responsible in fiscal decision making ■ Be responsible for completion of evaluation
Respect for People ■ Use informed consent ■ Maintain confidentiality ■ Maximize benefits and reduce harms	**Respect for People's Rights and Dignity** ■ Respecting others ■ Nondiscrimination ■ Exploitative relationships	**Respect for People** D1: Seek understanding of contextual elements of evaluation D2: Use current ethics and standards on informed consent and confidentiality	**Utility, Feasibility, Propriety, and Accuracy** U1: Audience identification (stakeholder identification) U3: Information scope and selection	**Integrity** ■ Be sensitive to cultural and social environment of all stakeholders

| Communicate respect for stakeholders | ■ Delegation to and supervision of subordinates
■ institutional approval
■ Informed consent
■ Incentives to participants
■ Deception in research
■ Interpretation and explanation of research and evaluation results
■ Privacy and confidentiality | D3: Maximize benefits and reduce harms from evaluation
D4: Communicate respect for stakeholders' dignity and self-worth
D5: Attempt to foster social equity in evaluation
D5: Understand and respect differences among participants | U4: Values identification (transparency of values)
U5: Report clarity (report comprehensiveness and clarity)
U6: Report timeliness and dissemination
U7: Evaluation impact (evaluation utilization and use)
F1: Practical procedures
F2: Political viability (diplomatic conduct)
P1: Service orientation
P3: Rights of human subjects (protection of individual rights)
P4: Human interactions
P6: Disclosure of findings
A10: Justified conclusions
A11: Impartial reporting | ■ Confer on contractual decisions such as: confidentiality, privacy |

Social Responsibility

■ Consider wider implications and side effects
■ Recognize obligations for public good

Concern for Others' Welfare and Social Responsibility

■ Seek to contribute to others' welfare
■ Are aware of their responsibilities to the community, the society in which they work, and the planet

Responsibilities for General and Public Welfare

E1: Include full range of stakeholders in planning and reporting
E2: Consider immediate outcomes as well as broad assumptions, implications, and potential side effects
E3: Allow stakeholders access to evaluation information
E4: Maintain balance between client needs and other needs
E5: Recognize obligations for public interest and good

contexts in which evaluators operate. One of those contexts includes organizational settings, and such standards provide a framework for the knowledge and skills needed by those undertaking evaluations within organizations.

Frameworks from Evaluation Texts

Textbooks used in teaching evaluation concepts and skills also provide a source for determining the knowledge and skills needed to undertake evaluations. Table 2.2 presents texts that have been selected because they deal with evaluations within an organizational context or they represent a particular perspective on evaluation. Together, these present a framework that identifies the knowledge and skills needed by those undertaking evaluations.

Unlike the previously reviewed evaluation standards, these texts identify some of the technical knowledge and skills needed by evaluators. Specifically, these texts discuss issues related to various evaluation theories, models, and approaches, certain types of research design, different types of data collection methods, and alternative data analysis options. These represent domains and competencies that can be useful to evaluators operating within organizational settings.

Content of Academic and Certificate Programs

Academic and certificate programs were selected for review, because they described competencies covered in their course or courses. The information from these various programs appears in Table 2.3. These academic and certificate programs, particularly that of the Evaluators' Institute, provide an overview of the content considered important for those who plan to practice evaluation.

TABLE 2.2   Comparison of the Contents of Books on Evaluation

Book Content Categories or Domains and Competencies	Basarab & Root (1992)	Owen & Rogers (1999)	Phillips (1997a, b)	Preskill & Russ-Eft (2005) and Russ-Eft & Preskill (2001)	Rossi, Freeman, & Lipsey (1999) and Rossi, Lipsey, & Freeman (2003)	Swanson & Holton (1999)
Understand evaluation background and history		Evaluation fundamentals Nature of interventions; what we evaluate	Understand the need for evaluation and measurement	Understand history of evaluation and training evaluation	Understand history	
Understand politics and use codes of ethics		Understand and use codes of behavior		Understand politics and ethics	Understand ethics, standards, and guidelines	
Understand multicultural and cross-cultural aspects				Understand multicultural and cross-cultural aspects	Tailor evaluations	

(Continued)

Book Content Categories or Domains and Competencies	Basarab & Root (1992)	Owen & Rogers (1999)	Phillips (1997a, b)	Preskill & Russ-Eft (2005) and Russ-Eft & Preskill (2001)	Rossi, Freeman, & Lipsey (1999) and Rossi, Lipsey, & Freeman (2003)	Swanson & Holton (1999)
Understand and use alternative evaluation models and approaches	Understand and use alternative evaluation models	Understand and use alternative evaluation models: Proactive Clarificative Interactive Monitoring Impact	Understand and use a results-based model: 1. Reaction 2. Testing 3. Skills and competencies Business results Evaluate outside resources	Understand and use alternative evaluation models: Behavioral objectives Responsive Expertise and accreditation Goal free Adversarial or judicial Consumer oriented Utilization focused Participatory or collaborative Empowerment Organizational learning Theory driven Success case	Understand and use alternative evaluation models: Program monitoring Impact assessment	Understand and use core concepts and models: Performance results: - Systems - Financial Learning results: - Knowledge and expertise Perception results: - Participants and stakeholders
Focus the evaluation		Focus the evaluation		Focus the evaluation	Identify issues and formulate questions Assess and express program theory	

Select an evaluation design	Develop appropriate evaluation design	Select an evaluation design	Understand and use randomized designs
			Understand and use nonrandomized designs
Develop appropriate data collection instruments and procedures; collect data	Develop data collection procedures: Observations Questionnaires Interviews Focus groups Tests Collect data	Design data collection instruments Collect evaluation data: Questionnaires Attitude surveys Participant feedback Tests Simulations Interviews Focus groups Observations Monitoring performance data Action planning Performance contracts	Choose data collection methods: Observations Archival data Questionnaires Interviews Focus groups	Collect data Critical outcome technique Auditing program practices and effectiveness Certification of core expertise Assessing performance drivers

(Continued)

Book Content Categories or Domains and Competencies	Basarab & Root (1992)	Owen & Rogers (1999)	Phillips (1997a, b)	Preskill & Russ-Eft (2005) and Russ-Eft & Preskill (2001)	Rossi, Freeman, & Lipsey (1999) and Rossi, Lipsey, & Freeman (2003)	Swanson & Holton (1999)
Select sample				Select sample		
Analyze data	Analyze data	Collect and analyze data: From evaluation questions to evaluation findings	Isolate effects of training Convert data to monetary benefits Identify intangible measures Determine program costs Analyze statistical data Determine return on investment	Analyze data: Qualitative Quantitative Cost-benefit; cost-effectiveness	Measure efficiency (cost-benefit, cost-effectiveness)	Measure results: Performance results: - Systems - Financial Learning results: - Knowledge and expertise Perception results: - Participants and stakeholders
Report progress and findings	Report results	Report results: From evaluation findings to utilization	Communicate program results	Communicate and report findings	Use evaluation results	Report assessment findings

	Plan the evaluation	Plan and negotiate the evaluation; determine key players and resources	Plan the implementation	Manage the evaluation	Plan results assessment
Plan, negotiate, and manage the evaluation	Plan the evaluation	Plan and negotiate the evaluation; determine key players and resources	Plan the implementation	Manage the evaluation	Plan results assessment
Evaluate the evaluation or metaevaluation	Measure effective evaluations (metaevaluation)			Evaluate the evaluation (metaevaluation)	
Build and sustain support for evaluation			Understand management influence on HRD program results	Build and sustain support	

Note: HRD = human resource development.

TABLE 2.3 Comparison of Academic and Certificate Programs in Evaluation

Program and Course Content or Domains and Competencies	Evaluators' Institute: Certificate in Evaluation Practice, Evaluation Methods	Fielding Institute: Certificate in Evaluation and Organizational Development	Florida State University: Master's, Doctorate, Certificate in Program Evaluation	Oregon State University: Master's in Adult Education	University of Melbourne: Master's, Doctorate, and Certificate in Assessment and Evaluation	University of Minnesota: Master's and Doctorate in Quantitative Methods in Education (QME) and in Educational Policy and Administration—Evaluation Studies Certificate in Educational Policy and Administration—Program Evaluation
Understand and use evaluation theories and models	Understand and use evaluation theories		Demonstrated knowledge in evaluation theory	Describe key models, theories, strategies	Understand, synthesize, and use key concepts and theories underlying policy and program development	
Understand multicultural issues	Understand multicultural issues					
Understand and use appropriate evaluation designs	Understand and use appropriate evaluation designs			Choose appropriate evaluation designs	Design the assessment or evaluation of programs	

Understand and use standards and ethics	Understand and use professional standards and ethics for evaluators		Describe standards and ethical practices	Act ethically and in accordance with recognized standards
Plan and manage evaluations, including communications, budget, and schedule	Manage evaluations Evaluation consulting business skills	Demonstrated knowledge in managing and implementing evaluations: Stakeholder identification Stakeholder communication Managing budget and schedule	Develop an evaluation plan	Manage the assessment or evaluation of programs; take leadership role in assessment and evaluation practice of high quality
Work with stakeholders to determine evaluation questions	Work with stakeholders Understand and use participatory or collaborative methods	Define organizational needs and goals Determine evaluation questions		

(Continued)

Program and Course Content or Domains and Competencies	Evaluators' Institute: Certificate in Evaluation Practice, Evaluation Methods	Fielding Institute: Certificate in Evaluation and Organizational Development	Florida State University: Master's, Doctorate, Certificate in Program Evaluation	Oregon State University: Master's in Adult Education	University of Melbourne: Master's, Doctorate, and Certificate in Assessment and Evaluation	University of Minnesota: Master's and Doctorate in Quantitative Methods in Education (QME) and in Educational Policy and Administration—Evaluation Studies Certificate in Educational Policy and Administration—Program Evaluation
Understand and use program theory or logic modeling	Understand and use program theory or logic modeling			Create logic model		
Understand and use various approaches and concepts: Needs assessment Product evaluation Process evaluation Performance measurement Outcome and impact evaluation	Understand and use various evaluation approaches: Needs assessment Process evaluation Performance measurement Outcome and impact evaluation Cost-benefit/cost-effectiveness analysis			Understand various evaluation concepts: Process evaluation Performance measurement Product evaluation Formative evaluation Summative evaluation Monitoring, auditing Outcome evaluation Impact evaluation	Understand and effectively use professional and scholarly literature in assessment and evaluation	

Cost-benefit/cost-effectiveness analysis	Policy evaluation	Internal and external evaluation	
Policy evaluation	Evaluability assessment		
Evaluability assessment			
Internal and external evaluation			
Understand and use appropriate quantitative methods	Understand and use applied statistics: Regression Meta-analysis Understand and use applied measurement	Measure organizational capacities, processes, and outcomes	Quantitative methods; statistical data analysis; computer database analysis
		Demonstrated skills in data analysis (compilation, entry, and analysis using statistical software)	
Understand and use appropriate qualitative methods	Understand and use qualitative inquiry methods and analysis		Qualitative inquiry
Select, design, and use appropriate data collection methods: **Observations** **Archival data** **Surveys** **Interviews** **Focus groups**	Design and administer surveys	Demonstrated knowledge of research methods: quantitative, qualitative, mixed methods	
		Choose appropriate data collection methods: Observations Archival data Surveys Interviews Focus groups Develop data collection tools	

(Continued)

Program and Course Content or Domains and Competencies	Evaluators' Institute: Certificate in Evaluation Practice, Evaluation Methods	Fielding Institute: Certificate in Evaluation and Organizational Development	Florida State University: Master's, Doctorate, Certificate in Program Evaluation	Oregon State University: Master's in Adult Education	University of Melbourne: Master's, Doctorate, and Certificate in Assessment and Evaluation	University of Minnesota: Master's and Doctorate in Quantitative Methods in Education (QME) and in Educational Policy and Administration—Evaluation Studies Certificate in Educational Policy and Administration—Program Evaluation
Understand and use appropriate sampling methods	Understand and use sampling					
Use appropriate analysis procedures	Link evaluation questions to analysis techniques			Choose appropriate analysis procedures		
Communicate and report results	Communicate and report results		Demonstrated competency in reporting evaluation outcomes	Determine communicating and reporting methods		Communication skills

	Ensure use of findings	Build organizational capacity for evaluation	Conduct a metaevaluation
Ensure use of findings	Use evaluation results for policy	Ensure use of findings	
Build organizational capacity for evaluation	Build organizational capacity for evaluation		Act as a resource for professional colleagues in assessment and evaluation situations
Conduct a metaevaluation		Conduct a metaevaluation	

Domains and Competencies Derived from Standards, Textbooks, and Programs

PROFESSIONAL FOUNDATIONS AND COMPETENCE

- Communicate accurately and effectively
- Observe ethical standards
- Obtain and maintain needed skills
- Understand evaluation background and history

PROFESSIONAL RESPONSIBILITY, INTEGRITY, ACCOUNTABILITY

- Accurately represent skills
- Disclose conflicts of interest
- Negotiate honestly
- Communicate accurately and fairly
- Understand politics

RESPECT FOR PEOPLE

- Use informed consent
- Maintain confidentiality
- Maximize benefits and reduce harms
- Communicate respect for stakeholders
- Understand multicultural and cross-cultural aspects

SOCIAL RESPONSIBILITY

- Consider wider implications and side effects
- Recognize obligations for public good

EVALUATION UNDERSTANDING AND PRACTICE

- Understand and use alternative evaluation theories, models, and approaches
- Focus the evaluation

- Work with stakeholders to determine evaluation questions

- Understand and use program theory or logic modeling

- Communicate and report progress and results

- Ensure use of findings

- Evaluate the evaluation *i.e.,* conduct metaevaluation

- Build and sustain support for evaluation *i.e.,* build organizational capacity for evaluation

RESEARCH SKILLS

- Develop or select an evaluation design

- Develop appropriate data collection instruments and procedures

- Use appropriate data collection methods

- Understand and use appropriate sampling methods

- Use appropriate qualitative and quantitative analysis procedures

PROJECT MANAGEMENT SKILLS

- Plan and negotiate the evaluation

- Develop plan for and manage communications

- Develop plan for and manage the budget

- Develop plan for and manage the schedule

Combined Results from Standards, Textbooks, and Programs

By taking all three sources together, we began to create a list of domains (or a grouping of competencies) and specific competencies that could be used in future research (see page 33, "Domains and Competencies Derived from Standards, Textbooks, and Programs").

Comparison with Evaluator-Generated Competencies

King et al. (2001) recognized that little work existed regarding competencies from the perspective of evaluation professionals, primarily those undertaking large-scale program evaluations. To do so, they conducted a Multi-Attribute Consensus Reaching (MARC) process with small groups of 3 to 10 individuals. A total of 31 professional evaluators or evaluation study students (3 men and 28 women) from the Minneapolis–St. Paul area participated in the study. The MARC process required participants to rate a set of evaluator competencies and then to discuss their rationale for the ratings. The sessions lasted approximately 2.5 hours. Because this work represents the only empirical study on evaluator competencies, we can compare the results from the three streams of literature with those from the King et al. work to identify the similarities and differences.

King et al. (2001) identified four domains and 65 competencies. The following list indicates the areas that appear in the King et al. work that do not emerge from the review of the various standards, book contents, and program syllabi. The items *not* in bold typeface represent those where the evaluators showed "real disagreement on perceived importance" (King et al., 2001, p. 235).

1. Conducts literature reviews

2. **Open to others' input**

3. **Able to adapt or change study as needed**

4. **Able to supervise others**

5. **Able to train others**

6. Able to conduct evaluation in nondisruptive manner

7. Able to deal with stress during a project

8. **Possesses negotiation skills**

9. Possesses conflict resolution skills

10. Possesses computer application skills

11. Possesses knowledge of self as an evaluator

12. Reflects on practice

13. Participates in networks

14. Contributes to the knowledge base of evaluation

Thus, of the four domains and 65 competencies identified by King et al. (2001), only 14 did not appear explicitly in the literature on evaluation standards, textbooks, and programs. Furthermore, of these 14, nine appeared to be in dispute among the small group of evaluators. These results provided some validation for the current effort. Critically needed next, however, was a more thorough and extensive validation effort.

CONCLUSIONS

Although greater emphasis and interest is emerging regarding evaluations within organizational settings, a comprehensive listing of the competencies needed for planning and conducting such evaluations does not currently exist, which validates the decision of ibstpi to undertake the development of standards for evaluators in organizational settings. In this chapter, we presented some initial work on competency development, highlighting existing sources from a variety of countries and contexts. The results can provide HRD professionals with validated evidence as to the needed competencies for undertaking evaluation efforts within their organizations. They will, however, need to be validated with those evaluators who work in organizational settings. In addition, the validation will need to take place within the global context. Such a validated competency model can then serve as the basis for developmental efforts aimed at improving the competencies of internal professionals as they undertake evaluation work within their own organizations. Furthermore, it can also serve those external evaluators who currently work or who plan to work within an organizational setting.

QUESTIONS FOR CONSIDERATION

How would you describe to someone what it means to be a "competent evaluator?"

What social, cultural, or operational factors might influence competencies important in your organization or in a particular organization?

CHAPTER

3

IBSTPI EVALUATOR COMPETENCIES AND THEIR DEVELOPMENT

This chapter will enable you to accomplish the following:

- Distinguish among the following concepts: competency, competence, competency model
- Identify and explain the structure of the ibstpi Evaluator Competency model
- Explain at least three assumptions of the ibstpi Evaluator Competencies

In this chapter, we focus on the conceptual and methodological frame underpinning the development of the ibstpi Evaluator Competencies. We start with a concise history of competency modeling, then briefly examine the context of the ibstpi competency development work and present the definition of competency used in this book. Readers will find a description of the generic ibstpi model used to develop the evaluator competencies as well as the underlying assumptions in the development and interpretation of the model. In the final section, we present the evaluator competencies model itself.

A BRIEF HISTORY OF COMPETENCY MODELING

Competency modeling refers to the process resulting in a cohesive description of human performance and the attributes of people required to perform effectively. That process yields a model—that is, an organized set of competencies and performance indicators. Some trace the first efforts in competency profiling to the early Romans in their attempts to describe the qualities of a "good Roman soldier" (Kierstead, 1998). However, given the various interpretations that the term *competency* has received, it would be difficult to find the roots of the competency modeling as we currently know it. Although Flanagan (1949, 1954), for example, never used the term competency, he nonetheless pioneered techniques to collecting data of observable behaviors of employees, objectively evaluating performance, and determining requirements of an activity. It is commonly agreed, though, that competency modeling was initiated in the late 1960s and early 1970s with research done by David McClelland (1973). That research introduced the concept of using competencies instead of academic aptitude or intelligence as an alternative way to measure and predict job performance, employee selection, and career development. More recently, the O*Net effort (National Center for O*NET Development, n.d.) resulted in defining a common dictionary for competencies that replaced the earlier Dictionary of Occupational Titles.

THE ibstpi COMPETENCY DEVELOPMENT MODEL

In the education field, the competency-based approach involved the application of tools and methods in assessing the effectiveness of teacher education programs (Dick, Watson, & Kaufman, 1981). Interest in the competency approach was also associated with the application of systems design techniques and elements of mastery learning to competency-based education (Dick, Carey, & Carey, 2004; Young & Van Mondfrans, 1972). It is in the context of this competency-based movement that the ibstpi work on competency models development is integrated.

The application of a competency-based approach can occur in many different settings, including academic or training settings, public and private sectors, and nonprofit and professional organizations. In light of this diversity of contexts and uses, it is not surprising that the nature of a competency and how it relates to professional competence itself can be viewed from different perspectives.

The Nature of Competence and Competencies

The competency construct has been conceptualized in many ways (Catano, 1998; Le Boterf, 2001; Spencer & Spencer, 1993; Toolsema, 2003). Most of the definitions of competency focus on knowledge, skills, and attitudes as main components of competencies (Hooghiemstra, 1992; Lucia & Lepsinger, 1999; McLagan, 1997; Parry, 1998). A major divergent viewpoint exists concerning the personality traits, qualities, and values. According to Parry (1998), some mistake these personal attributes for the nature of competencies, instead of including them as foundational to skill and knowledge demonstration. Similarly, the terms *competence* and *competency* are sometimes equated (Van Merriënboer, Van der Klink, & Hendriks, 2002). However, some authors argue that there is a distinction between the two concepts (Klein, 1996; Rowe, 1995; Woodruff, 1991). For Richey, Fields, and Foxon (2001), competence and competency are different but interrelated concepts: competence refers to the state of being well qualified, and a competency describes the critical ways in which competence is demonstrated. In that context, ibstpi defines a competency as "a set of related knowledge, skills, and attitudes that enable an individual to effectively perform the activities of a given occupation or job function to the standards expected in employment" (Richey, Fields, & Foxon, 2001, p. 31).

The ibstpi definition includes two approaches to competency identified by McLagan (1997), namely the association of competencies with performance on a job and the use of knowledge, skills, and attitudes as main foundations of effective performance. It also implies that the knowledge, skills, and attitudes can be measured against commonly accepted standards. This perspective places emphasis on the competencies as statements of performance, rather than as personality traits or specific personal attributes that cannot be changed. The implication, therefore, is that the ibstpi competencies can be developed through training. However, an evaluator may be asked to evaluate whether an intervention that addresses unchangeable attributes of people achieved its objectives. This could include, for example, evaluating whether a new prehire selection process effectively predicts job performance without discriminating against various groups (e.g., women, minorities) and before employing and training those individuals.

The ibstpi Generic Competency Development Model

The set of competencies for a defined occupation or organizational role, such as the ibstpi Evaluator Competencies, can be represented in a competency model. According to Marrelli (1998), a competency model refers to "the organization of identified competencies into a conceptual framework that enables the people in an organization to understand, talk about, and apply the competencies" (p. 10). Another definition specifies that a competency model "represent[s] the most critical knowledge, skills, and behaviors that drive successful performance with respect to a particular type of job or occupation, . . . competencies in behavioral terms, . . . and behavioral indicators, so employees can recognize the competencies when demonstrated" (HR [Human Resources] Guide to the Internet, 2000, para. 1). Thus, a competency model gives structure to a collection of competencies by organizing the knowledge, skills, and attitudes using a specific framework. Furthermore, it includes performance indicators that describe how each competency is demonstrated in a job context.

To build a competency model effectively, ibstpi uses a generic competency development model that leverages input from several levels of analysis in order to define each competency. The model puts in perspective the link between the competencies, the job role, and how each competency is demonstrated. (An analogous interpretation of a competency model in an organizational context is proposed by Hendry and Maggio [1996], suggesting that it also denotes the relation of the competencies with the broader goals of an organization.) Figure 3.1 provides a graphic representation of the ibstpi competency model.

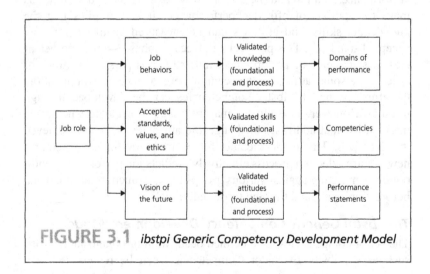

FIGURE 3.1 *ibstpi Generic Competency Development Model*

The first level, the definition of the job role, dictates the major orientations and scope of the competency model. Defining the role tends to be a preliminary step to competency definition. For example, a role can be defined in a generic way or be customized or specific to a job context (Lucia & Lepsinger, 1999). The approach used in the ibstpi Evaluator Competencies corresponds to a generalized view of the evaluator's role but specifically oriented toward that role as focused on evaluations within the organization. According to their particular positions, different evaluators may require only certain competencies of the model. Indeed, it is highly unlikely that an evaluator will need all of the competencies at any one time, but these competencies will emerge over the course of different evaluations done in different settings.

The job roles must be interpreted further to facilitate competency definition. At this second level of the development, specific behaviors that are characteristic of the evaluator are identified. For example, an important behavior for an evaluator involves collecting data on the program, process, or product to be evaluated. It is also important to determine the standards of performance associated with the identified behaviors as well as the professional values and ethics prevailing in the field. Thus, in collecting data, the evaluator should follow certain standards to ensure accuracy in the data collection and certain ethical guidelines to ensure confidentiality of the data. To complete this level of analysis, it is essential to distinguish the vision that gives shape and direction to the evaluator's role. "This vision may be the result of interpretations of current research and emerging trends, or it may be the result of societal or business pressures" (Foxon et al., 2003, p. 24).

A major issue at this stage of the analysis is balancing what appears as current practice with what ibstpi and our expert advisors believe the role is or should be. It is the tension between *what is* and *what should be*. An analysis of trends, expectations, and future vision of how the evaluator role will develop over the next five to ten years influences the analysis. For example, ibstpi sees a trend toward more outsourcing, and this has led to the inclusion of a performance statement about managing consultants.

The information gathered on behaviors, standards, ethics, values, and vision of a job role guide the third level of analysis that results in the identification of knowledge, skills, and attitudes required by evaluators. Finally, at the fourth level, this information is organized according to three components: domains, competencies, and performance statements.

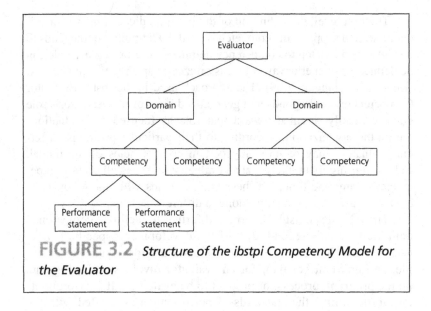

FIGURE 3.2 *Structure of the ibstpi Competency Model for the Evaluator*

Figure 3.2 represents the organization of the knowledge, skills, and attitudes according to the structure of the ibstpi model.

Domains are clusters of related competencies. This categorization serves to establish the relationship between competencies according to larger areas of activities. In the ibstpi Evaluator Competency model, the competencies have been grouped in four domains: professional foundations, planning and designing the evaluation, implementing the evaluation plan, and managing the evaluation.

Competencies are the core component of the ibstpi model. They are short statements, each one providing a general description of a complex effort. The managing and evaluation domain, for example, encompasses two competencies: monitor the management plan and work effectively with personnel and stakeholders.

Each competency is supported by a list of performance statements that provide a fuller description of how it is demonstrated. For example, the performance statements supporting the competency Managing the Evaluation include Adapt the plan to meet changing circumstances and Track evaluation progress against schedule. The performance statements are not procedural steps but, rather, elaborations of the competency statement in behavioral and measurable terms.

Implementing the Model for Evaluators

The ibstpi competency development model is the key driver of the competency development process used to develop diverse job role competency models, including Instructional Designer (Richey, Fields, & Foxon, 2001), Training Manager (Foxon et al., 2003), and Instructor (Klein et al., 2004). Operationally, it can be summed up by three phases, each of which is fundamentally an empirical procedure:

▪ *Phase 1. Identification of foundational research.* The foundation of the ibstpi Evaluator Competency model was based on an extensive review of programs, courses, and training modules in evaluation provided by universities and evaluation associations around the world.

▪ *Phase 2. Competency drafting.* The base list of competencies was analyzed and debated by ibstpi members, with particular expertise in different areas of evaluation. In addition, experts in evaluation reviewed and commented on these drafts.

▪ *Phase 3. Competency validation and rewriting.* A validation instrument was designed, developed, pilot tested, and administered worldwide via the web. The results and statements were submitted to the entire ibstpi membership to ensure coherence with the board's mission, vision, and values. Details on the entire process for the Evaluator Competency validation process can be found in Chapters 6 and 7.

ASSUMPTIONS UNDERLYING THE IBSTPI EVALUATOR COMPETENCIES

The ibstpi Evaluator Competencies are based on some general assumptions that are critical to understanding the competencies and their use.

Assumption 1. Evaluators are persons who demonstrate evaluator competencies on the job regardless of their job title or training.

Even though most experienced evaluators take it for granted that people are clear as to who evaluators are, in some cases that distinction may not be completely obvious. Those undertaking evaluations within organizational settings, in most cases, do not possess a job title indicating the role of evaluator. Certainly many who undertake evaluations within organizational settings have acquired their skills on the job or by attending short workshops, rather than by completing formal academic programs and earning a degree. Nevertheless, these competencies are relevant to all of those individuals.

Assumption 2. ibstpi Evaluator Competencies pertain to evaluators working in a wide range of job settings.

ibstpi competencies are built to be universally applicable, but they are not meant to cover all possible applications. An evaluator role can be performed in a variety of settings, and the scope of the competencies model needs to be clarified. However, the competencies included in the model presented in this book target evaluators working within organizational settings, including for-profit and not-for-profit organizations, the military, and government agencies evaluating their own internal programs. These competencies may or may not be applicable to those undertaking evaluations of large-scale government-funded programs.

Assumption 3. ibstpi Evaluator Competencies define the manner in which an evaluator job role should be practiced.

More than reflecting current practice of a job role, ibstpi competencies represent professional standards expected to be upheld by that role. By following a systematic development process, including a thorough validation, the Evaluator Competencies model explicitly describes the knowledge, skills, and attitudes expected of an evaluator. In a sense, the model serves as a benchmark for the way the evaluator practice should be practiced.

Assumption 4. Evaluation is a process most commonly guided by systematic models and principles.

As described in Chapter 1, various models and approaches are used in conducting evaluations. Although ibstpi does not ascribe to any one specific approach or model, the ibstpi Evaluator Competencies are firmly rooted in a belief that evaluation is, and should be, practiced using one or more of the systematic models or approaches.

Assumption 5. ibstpi Evaluator Competencies span novice and experienced evaluators.

The ibstpi competencies were designed to be relevant to all levels of expertise. Although the validation did not focus on identifying different levels of expertise and their relevance, these competencies are important for all evaluators working within organizational settings.

Assumption 6. ibstpi Evaluator Competencies should be meaningful and useful worldwide.

Evaluation is a job role practiced all around the world. Even though particular aspects of the evaluator role vary, and certain terms may differ from country to country, there are nonetheless overarching principles and commonalities that are critical to all. To reach international use of the Evaluator Competencies, resources around the world were involved in the competency development and validation processes, taking care to ensure international input.

Assumption 7. ibstpi Evaluator Competencies are generic and amenable to customization.

The application of ibstpi competencies is broad. Because the evaluator competencies are written to be as inclusive as possible, it is expected that they will be used as a standard for evaluators within organizational settings. To be put to use in actual work environments, the competencies may be adapted to blend into the particular characteristics of the culture of the environment. For example, although all evaluators are expected to observe ethical and legal standards, the conditions governing that competency may be different according to a particular organization or evaluation project.

Assumption 8. ibstpi Evaluator Competencies reflect societal and disciplinary values and ethics.

The ibstpi competencies reflect trends, emerging issues, and particular philosophies of the times in which the specific model is built. Thus, the Evaluator Competencies model suggests certain positions about the evaluation field, reflecting a time in which the evaluator's role is permeated by trends and issues including, among others, gender, globalization, cultural diversity, accountability, and human rights. The sociocultural changes and evolution in the evaluation field have an impact on the evaluator's role and thus in the competencies model, reflecting the dynamism of the profession.

CONCLUSIONS

Competency modeling provides a method for determining the critical skills, knowledge, abilities, and attitudes needed for a particular job. The ibstpi approach to competency modeling examines the job behaviors; the accepted standards, values, and ethics; and the vision of the future. It then takes the resulting domains, competencies, and performance statements and validates them with those persons who are actually performing the particular job. Thus, such an approach, as used with the ibstpi Evaluator Competencies, yields a model that reflects the evaluator job role both today and in the future. The ibstpi Evaluator Competencies model can be found in the box at the end of this chapter.

QUESTIONS FOR CONSIDERATION

What makes a competency model an authoritative tool for you or others?

What are the differences among the concepts of competence, competency, and competency model? Why might these differences be important?

The 2006 ibstpi Evaluator Domains, Competencies, and Performance Statements*

The 2006 evaluator competencies developed by ibstpi include 14 competencies clustered in four general domains and supported by 84 performance statements. These are competencies required by internal staff or external consultants conducting evaluations in organizational settings, such as for-profit and not-for-profit organizations, military, and government agencies evaluating their own internal programs. The competencies required by such individuals are different from those required by evaluators examining the effectiveness of large-scale statewide or national programs often funded by government departments or agencies. Competencies for such large-scale evaluations are provided by professional evaluation associations, such as the American Evaluation Association and the Canadian Evaluation Society, and are covered in numerous textbooks on program evaluation.

They reflect the core competencies of evaluators in these organizational settings—the skills, knowledge, and attitudes that a competent evaluator must demonstrate to successfully complete an evaluation assignment within an organization.

Professional Foundations

1. Communicate effectively in written, oral, and visual form.

   a. Use verbal and nonverbal language appropriate to the audience, context, and culture.

   b. Use active listening skills.

   c. Choose appropriate technology to enhance communication.

   d. Simplify and summarize complex information.

   e. Facilitate meetings effectively.

   f. Demonstrate effective presentation skills.

   g. Write clearly and concisely.

2. Establish and maintain professional credibility.

   a. Model exemplary professional conduct.

   b. Demonstrate relevant organizational, business, and industry knowledge.

   c. Stay current with new thinking and approaches in evaluation and related fields.

   d. Update one's professional skills.

   e. Stay current with relevant technology.

   f. Participate in professional activities related to evaluation.

   g. Share knowledge and experience to develop evaluation skills in others.

   h. Document one's work as a foundation for future efforts, professional presentations, or publication.

   i. Establish and maintain professional networks.

3. Demonstrate effective interpersonal skills.

   a. Be sensitive to cultural norms and organizational practices.

   b. Establish and maintain effective working relationships.

   c. Use consulting skills to clarify issues.

   d. Use negotiation skills.

   e. Use conflict resolution skills.

   f. Monitor and respond to the dynamics of groups and teams.

(Continued)

4. Observe ethical and legal standards.

   a. Comply with organizational and professional codes of ethics.

   b. Comply with applicable laws and regulations.

   c. Respect the need for confidentiality and anonymity.

   d. Declare or avoid conflicts of interest.

   e. Respect intellectual property including proprietary rights.

5. Demonstrate awareness of the politics of evaluation.

   a. Identify the potential political implications of each evaluation.

   b. Clarify stakeholder values.

   c. Attend to political issues as they arise.

Planning and Designing the Evaluation

6. Develop an effective evaluation plan.

   a. Describe the program, process, or product to be evaluated.

   b. Identify the stakeholders.

   c. Identify the evaluation focus and key questions to be answered.

   d. Use best practices or relevant literature to guide the evaluation plan.

   e. Describe the evaluation strategy and expected outcomes.

   f. Identify models, methods, or designs to support the evaluation.

   g. Collaborate with stakeholders to confirm the selected approach and evaluation design.

7. Develop a management plan for the evaluation.

   a. Develop the evaluation schedule, responsibilities, and deliverables.

   b. Determine the budget.

   c. Identify internal and external personnel requirements.

   d. Determine training needs of personnel.

   e. Determine technology requirements.

   f. Allocate personnel and resources to support the plan.

   g. Develop a communication and reporting plan.

   h. Obtain needed permissions regarding confidentiality.

   i. Prepare and negotiate a proposal.

8. Devise data collection strategies to support the evaluation questions and design.

   a. Identify potential data sources.

   b. Draw on a variety of evaluation instruments and procedures.

   c. Evaluate the appropriateness of using existing instruments and tools.

   d. Construct reliable and valid instruments.

   e. Develop a data collection plan, including protocols and procedures.

   f. Design appropriate sampling procedures.

   g. Address threats to trustworthiness and validity of data.

   h. Develop a plan for data analysis and interpretation.

   i. Plan for the storage, security, and disposal of data.

9. Pilot test the data collection instruments and procedures.

   a. Design the pilot test.

   b. Identify an appropriate sample.

   c. Implement changes based on feedback and results.

Implementing the Evaluation Plan

10. Collect data.

   a. Implement the data collection plan, schedule, and budget.

   b. Document evaluation activities.

   c. Conduct effective individual or group interviews.

   d. Conduct effective observations.

   e. Record and summarize relevant existing data.

   f. Respond to changes in the scope or focus of the evaluation.

   g. Minimize disruptions during data collection.

11. Analyze and interpret data.

   a. Assess the trustworthiness, validity, and reliability of data.

   b. Use appropriate quantitative or qualitative analysis procedures.

   c. Review and interpret data in an unbiased way.

(Continued)

    d. Make judgments about the findings and draw conclusions.

    e. Develop recommendations.

12. Disseminate and follow up the findings and recommendations.

    a. Use multiple methods of communicating and reporting.

    b. Discuss and interpret the evaluation findings with stakeholders.

    c. Present the findings according to the needs of diverse audiences.

    d. Facilitate or monitor changes resulting from recommendations.

Managing the Evaluation

13. Monitor the management plan.

    a. Adapt the plan to meet changing circumstances.

    b. Review and adjust the budget, if needed.

    c. Track evaluation progress against schedule.

    d. Identify and resolve problems that arise during the evaluation.

    e. Foster reflection and dialogue on the evaluation process and outcomes.

14. Work effectively with personnel and stakeholders.

    a. Manage team members, consultants, and technical experts.

    b. Keep stakeholders informed of progress.

    c. Keep the evaluation team engaged in and informed of the progress.

    d. Debrief evaluation team and stakeholders to establish lessons learned.

    e. Assess stakeholder satisfaction with the evaluation.

CHAPTER

DISCUSSION AND ANALYSIS OF THE EVALUATOR DOMAINS AND COMPETENCIES

This chapter will enable you to accomplish the following:

- Describe the structure of the ibstpi Evaluator Competency model in terms of domains, competencies, and performance statements

- Identify domains critical for evaluators

- Identify competencies critical for evaluators

- Identify performance statements relevant for evaluators looking to keep up to date in the field

- Describe how a prospective evaluator can use the competency model to orient his or her career

- Outline a portfolio that will showcase personal proficiency in the professional foundations domain

In this chapter, we explore the dimensions of the domains and competencies identified for evaluators. We describe each of the four domains—*Professional Foundations, Planning and Designing the Evaluation, Implementing the Evaluation Plan,* and *Managing the Evaluation*—and discuss their associated competencies and performance statements.

PROFESSIONAL FOUNDATIONS

The first competency domain for evaluators is *Professional Foundations,* and it pertains to five competency areas:

- Communications
- Professional credibility
- Interpersonal skills
- Ethical and legal standards
- Politics of evaluation

This competency domain is an explicit recognition of the professional status of evaluation specialists, and it represents a domain that appears in each of the other ibstpi competency frameworks: training manager, instructional designer, and instructor. As with any profession, evaluation specialists have an obligation to communicate clearly and coherently with and to stakeholders and the evaluation community at large. Because of the complex process of evaluation, it is important for evaluators to establish credibility and maintain effective evaluation practices. They should also actively engage in advancing the evaluation profession and work effectively with diverse groups of stakeholders in dynamic environments. Given the sensitive nature of evaluative data and the potential impact of evaluation results, evaluators are also obligated to maintain ethical practices, operate within legal guidelines, and demonstrate an awareness of the political implications of all aspects of the evaluation process.

The competency and associated performance statements are outlined below, accompanied by further discussion and explanation.

1. Communicate effectively in written, oral, and visual form. This competency includes the following seven performance standards:

a) Use verbal and nonverbal language appropriate to the audience, context, and culture.

b) Use active listening skills.

c) Choose appropriate technology to enhance communication.

d) Simplify and summarize complex information.

e) Facilitate meetings effectively.

f) Demonstrate effective presentation skills.

g) Write clearly and concisely.

The role of effective communication is emphasized in this set of standards. Evaluation practices are highly dependent on observing verbal and nonverbal expressions, listening attentively to others to effectively receive and interpret information. They also include facilitating communications among individuals and groups and communicating clearly and concisely in written form.

This competency is perhaps one of the most important to competent evaluation specialists. Communications permeates all tasks and activities in the evaluation process. Evaluation is in part about gathering, interpreting, and reporting data on the level of satisfaction, learning, performance, or impact that should be achieved. Evaluation is also about identifying issues concerning a program, a process, or a product and determining what modifications can be made to resolve such issues. As such, evaluators must possess the communication competencies to articulate accurately and persuasively the expected and achieved satisfaction, learning, and performance levels as well as the program, process, or product issues and solutions. This requires effective questioning and active listening proficiencies, accomplished presentation skills, and clear writing abilities that are acceptable and culturally sensitive to the audience within the evaluation context.

Effective communicators send and receive messages through both verbal and nonverbal signals and understand the implications of these signals within the context and culture of their audience. For example, facial expressions, certain terminology, and body gestures can signify vastly different messages to distinct cultures or organizations. Observing and inquiring into such signals are essential to accurate interpretation of evaluation data. Such skills are needed not only for interactions with the client and stakeholders but also when conducting individual interviews or focus groups.

Communicating effectively also requires strong active listening skills. This means listening to others in a way that focuses entirely on what they are saying and confirming understanding of both the content of the message and the emotions and feelings underlying the message to ensure that understanding is accurate. Good active listening requires effective questioning skills to prompt for clarity and validate interpretation of communication interactions.

Competent evaluators are able to effectively choose appropriate technologies that will facilitate communication and reception of evaluation information. Different types of technologies can be effective in gathering different types of information. For example, on one extreme, an evaluator who is interested in gathering objective evaluative ratings from a large population highly connected and communicative through electronic means may choose to communicate through Internet-based surveys (such as Zoomerang; available at http://info.zoomerang.com) or e-mail (through in-house distribution networks). On another extreme, an evaluator who is looking for thoughts and feelings from people who are diverse in their attitudes toward a program being evaluated and unable to meet in person to describe their thoughts may choose to use videoconferencing technologies to interview individuals or groups of participants. This technology may be an appropriate, efficient, and cost-effective method to gather both verbal and nonverbal feedback. Knowledge of available technologies and their uses for data collection, analysis, and communication can facilitate efficient and effective communication processes. Given the globalization of many organizations, most evaluators will need to become increasingly proficient in the use of electronic technology to conduct all phases of an evaluation, but particularly the data collection.

Communication skills require the ability to simplify and summarize complex information throughout the evaluation. Such complex information can come from interactions and meetings with the clients and stakeholders to determine the design and plan for the evaluation. This complex information also comes from the data collection and analysis undertaken as key elements of any evaluation, and these competencies are described in greater detail later in this chapter. Indeed, so much of what an evaluator captures, particularly in interviews and focus groups but also in surveys and document reviews, can prove to be difficult to reduce to something readable and easily understood. At the same time, such summarization needs to avoid losing the key nuances that yield critical details and that affect the clarity of the findings.

Another area of concern with regard to communications involves facilitating the many meetings required. Such meetings may include those with a client team (where the goal is to gain the background context needed to begin the evaluation effort), with stakeholders who want to have input in how the evaluation is done, with participants to gather needed information, and with the evaluation team members to plan the next steps. Meetings enable the evaluator to gather needed data, exchange ideas, and present information on the evaluation's progress and findings. An effective meeting facilitator or leader begins with clear goals and an agenda in mind; depending on the formality of the meeting, these goals and agenda may or may not be presented. Meeting leadership also requires skills in active listening, discussion facilitation, and conflict resolution. There is, in addition, a need to remain flexible and to change the agenda as the situation demands. Such skills help to keep any meeting on track and lead to agreed-on decisions and action plans.

Finally, effective evaluators demonstrate competencies in both presentation and writing skills. As discussed in later sections, the evaluator must present and write about progress and findings concerning the evaluation. Thus, an evaluator must demonstrate competence in presenting essential information clearly and precisely, organizing information logically, creating messages appropriate to an audience, using visual and written representations meaningfully and effectively, and responding to questions that arise, both in written and verbal forms. Technical writing, message design, and digital and visual literacy skills are a few of the supportive areas where evaluators should show competence.

2. *Establish and maintain professional credibility.* This competency includes the following nine performance standards:

a) Model exemplary professional conduct.

b) Demonstrate relevant organizational, business, and industry knowledge.

c) Stay current with new thinking and approaches in evaluation and related fields.

d) Update one's professional skills.

e) Stay current with relevant technology.

f) Participate in professional activities related to evaluation.

g) Share knowledge and experience to develop evaluation skills in others.

h) Document one's work as a foundation for future efforts, professional presentations, or publication.

i) Establish and maintain professional networks.

This competency is focused on both gaining and maintaining credibility with clients, stakeholders, evaluation team members, participants, organization members, and other evaluation professionals. Only through such credibility can an evaluator earn the needed trust to evaluate some program, process, or product.

At a basic level, the effective evaluator models exemplary professional conduct. This means that the evaluator recognizes that any and all conduct during the evaluation will come under scrutiny. In the course of the work, participants and respondents will describe what they think and feel, and such discussions and descriptions not only may influence the program, process, or product but also may affect people's careers. Furthermore, in modeling exemplary conduct, the evaluator serves as a role model for others within the organization and on the evaluation team. Finally, modeling professional conduct suggests attention to competency 4, focused on observing ethical and legal standards.

For evaluators within organizational settings, it is critical to demonstrate relevant organizational, business, and industry knowledge. Evaluation is more than just going into an organization and administering a survey or conducting interviews and analyzing data. An evaluator needs to understand the focus of the organization, its culture and its values, and the relationship of the program being evaluated to those elements. An evaluator's credibility is dependent on the ability to demonstrate a good understanding of the organization, its mission, and its people. Such an evaluator can increase stakeholder and participant trust in that evaluator and the work. This applies even for those who are internal to the organization. When undertaking an evaluation of a particular program, process, or product, an effective evaluator will obtain as much advance information as possible concerning the organization and its mission as well as the industry or business sector. In some cases, such data collection may also need to encompass information about the geographic region and the regulatory environment. When meeting with the client, stakeholders, and participants, the effective evaluator should be prepared to discuss these organizational conditions and to describe previous experiences undertaking evaluation or data collection efforts in similar organizations and circumstances.

Credibility can also be achieved through developing and updating professional evaluation skills and knowledge and through sharing that knowledge and experience with others. Knowledge of research and developments in evaluation practices, techniques, instruments, and technologies and their application should be a high priority for anyone undertaking an evaluation within an organization. As such, an effective evaluator should feel comfortable reading and interpreting both quantitative and qualitative research of evaluation studies and should routinely read about the latest research on evaluation methods, models, and practices. To enhance his or her credibility, an effective evaluator will then use this knowledge to inform clients and stakeholders and to discuss the various alternatives that may be used in the proposed evaluation. This discussion should include a description of both the benefits and the limitations to each of the suggested alternatives.

One aspect of knowledge development especially critical for today's evaluators is digital technologies. This involves learning about new technologies and their use in expediting evaluation processes, collecting data for an evaluation, supporting accurate data analyses, and facilitating effective and efficient communication among evaluation stakeholders. It is incumbent on evaluators to explore the available technologies, including computer-adaptive technologies that can be used within a particular organization for communication, data collection, and data analysis.

Participation in professional activities and professional organizations is key to becoming recognized as a credible evaluator. Such participation provides the opportunity to learn about the latest developments, whether these are related to evaluation, technology, or some particular organizational issues. Furthermore, this participation need not be simply focused on gaining additional knowledge and skills. It may also provide a means for sharing reflections on one's work. Such reflection and documentation can then be used for future projects and for presentation and publication in professional venues, and they are critical to advancing the field as well as an individual's professional skills. Some professional associations that can aid evaluators in such knowledge sharing are listed in Appendix E.

Sharing knowledge and experience does not only occur within professional associations but can also take place within an organization. It is important to share with others in an organization who are new to evaluation. To some degree, the more experienced evaluator has an obligation to build capability in an organization.

Throughout any evaluation, the evaluator must be scrupulous in documenting work. It is critical to keep field notes, meeting notes, working papers, and other files so that others can access them when needed. Furthermore, such documentation can reduce time later in the project, particularly when having to prepare final reports. Finally, maintaining such documents can aid in future work because it will facilitate the reuse of surveys or protocols as well as specific processes.

Involvement in professional associations and sharing one's knowledge and experience within the organization also aid in establishing a network. Through professional associations and their conferences and professional development seminars, evaluators meet others who are undertaking similar measurement efforts. There may be opportunities to meet authors of relevant articles or books. Sharing within the organization brings evaluators into contact and close communication with staff members possessing a wide range of skills and experiences, some of which may prove helpful to the evaluators. Such interactions and meetings can enable evaluators to contact knowledgeable individuals concerning specific questions or issues and may yield tools or ideas that can be used in an evaluation effort.

3. Demonstrate effective interpersonal skills. This competency includes the following six performance standards:

a) Be sensitive to cultural norms and organizational practices.

b) Establish and maintain effective working relationships.

c) Use consulting skills to clarify issues.

d) Use negotiation skills.

e) Use conflict resolution skills.

f) Monitor and respond to the dynamics of groups and teams.

A competent evaluator has effective and dynamic interpersonal skills that demonstrate sensitivity to the cultural and business practices of different groups participating in the evaluation. Clearly evaluators must be aware of and able to respond appropriately to cultural differences when working in a country or culture group different from their own. Western evaluators working in Asia, for example, need to be sensitive to the different ways and time frames of establishing rapport, conducting meetings, and so on. Similarly, the way in which agendas and time lines are viewed can vary from one culture to another and cause considerable frustration for evaluators who expect that the attitude to time is the same in every country!

Organizations also have their own cultural norms and include such elements as beliefs, habits, values, and rituals. For example, one organization may have an open culture where everyone is encouraged to say what they think, no matter who is in the room. The culture of another organization may be quite different; employees tend to keep what they think to themselves, especially if anyone from the management level is present. It is easy to see, therefore, how organizational culture can affect data collection when working with groups or individuals.

Organizational practices, on the other hand, refer to accepted operational practices in an organization—for example, knowing who should be consulted or invited to meetings, when and how information should be distributed, and who should be copied on what. Even within organizations, cultural practices can vary from one business group to another.

Evaluators must establish and maintain effective working relationships with a variety of stakeholders. These stakeholders include the client and primary stakeholder as well as others within the organization. The other stakeholders can include senior management, middle management, human resources (HR) and HR development staff, supervisory personnel, and frontline workers. An evaluation of a program, process, or product can involve and affect all levels within an organization. Only by establishing a good relationship with all of these different types of individuals will an evaluator be able to undertake needed data collection, whether that data collection involves document reviews, observations, surveys, interviews, or focus groups.

Whether an evaluator works inside an organization as an employee or is hired for a project as an external consultant, each needs a high level of consulting skill. Internal employees sometimes fail to see their role as that of a consultant. Typical consulting skills include the ability to gain a clear understanding from the primary stakeholders about what they want (and whether it is doable in terms of allocated time and resources), summarize feedback, negotiate a budget, arrive at a clear understanding on the process and time line, resolve conflicts or differences of opinion on how aspects of the evaluation should be conducted, and respond to both positive and negative dynamics of groups and teams. Evaluators may also play multiple roles such as team communicator, interpreter, coach or mentor, mediator, and decision maker, all of which require interpersonal skills, competencies, and sensitivity to other opinions and needs.

Negotiation skills are important because almost all aspects of an evaluation need to be negotiated with various stakeholders. An external evaluator will need to negotiate with the client for the resources and the budget for the evaluation and, in some cases, so will an internal evaluator. In addition, the evaluation plan and activities, the schedule for the data collection, and the people from whom data will be collected represent some of the aspects of an evaluation that will need to be negotiated by almost all evaluators. An evaluator must be able to communicate requirements as well as collaborate and reach consensus to achieve the goals and objectives of the evaluation.

In some instances, an evaluator will need to employ conflict resolution skills. These may be required when conflicts occur between various stakeholders. In the case of a larger evaluation effort, these skills may be needed to resolve conflicts among team members. In both cases, the evaluator must be able to maintain a neutral, objective stance; by doing so, he or she may help the opposing sides recognize other viewpoints and come to some areas of agreement and compromise.

Because an evaluator is working within an organizational setting, that person must be able to monitor and respond to dynamics of groups and teams. These dynamics may arise in the above-mentioned instances in which negotiation and conflict resolution skills may be needed. But these dynamics can also occur during meetings with the client and with stakeholder groups. Furthermore, conducting observations, interviews, and focus groups can bring the evaluator into situations in which it will be important to monitor group or team dynamics.

4. *Observe ethical and legal standards.* This competency includes the following five performance standards:

a) Comply with organizational and professional codes of ethics.

b) Comply with applicable laws and regulations.

c) Respect the need for confidentiality and anonymity.

d) Declare or avoid conflicts of interest.

e) Respect intellectual property, including proprietary rights.

As with any professional practice, evaluators have ethical and legal obligations. This competency is essential because evaluators are frequently dealing with sensitive data on personnel and performance. In addition, evaluators consulting inside an organization must review proprietary information. Organizations generally have codes of ethics, nondisclosure rules and agreements, and guidelines regarding the protection of personal information. Evaluators have a responsibility to be completely familiar with these ethical and legal requirements and to be scrupulous in compliance.

It should be recognized that engaging in ethical practices and following established legal standards also maintain evaluators' professional credibility. Some existing professional ethical practice guidelines, for example, advocate that evaluators display honesty and integrity in their behavior and work to ensure the honesty and integrity of the entire evaluation process (American Evaluation Association, 2004). Such practices help to ensure the credibility of the evaluator and the evaluation findings. Furthermore, the ethical guidelines and standards also recommend that evaluators protect privacy, prevent deception, and avoid conflicts related to their role as reporter, manager, objective scientist, and member of a profession (Newman & Brown, 1996). Chapter 1 introduces some of the ethical guidelines and standards, and Chapter 6 provides more details on several of these.

Maintaining confidentiality throughout the conduct of an evaluation is critical and something that a novice may not understand well enough. As an example, an internal contact, in wanting to help the external evaluator succeed, might suggest getting the vice president to "lean on" selected respondents by sending them an e-mail asking them to make the time available for an interview. Although sounding attractive, this may actually breach a promise of complete anonymity because the e-mail would mean that the vice president knew who had been selected for the interviews and could then make various assumptions about their responses.

The following are some suggestions for maintaining confidentiality in the conduct of an evaluation. The evaluator should be explicit in a covering e-mail or letter for a survey as to who will see the information and whether the respondents' names or e-mail addresses will be known. The same should be stated for individual interviews and focus groups; participants should be notified as to how the results will be presented and what level of confidentiality and anonymity will be provided. Once such guidelines are established, they should be strictly followed. The evaluator should not divulge confidential information, even if pressured by senior management. When writing up "stories" from interviews, the evaluator should ensure that they are sufficiently camouflaged that the source cannot be identified, even when the stories are positive ones. In addition, when reporting stories, the evaluator should ask respondents if they want to review drafts and read what has been written before it goes into the evaluation report to ensure it sufficiently protects their identity.

It is also important that evaluators declare or completely avoid conflicts of interest between the evaluation work in which they are engaged and personal interests in programs, personnel, or outside organizations. An evaluator should consider the ethics involved in agreeing to evaluate a vendor-provided program if, for example, the spouse works for that vendor company. It could be argued that this relationship compromises the evaluator's ability to give an unbiased evaluation of the program.

A final area of concern involves respecting intellectual property rights. It may be that an evaluator will want to use some tool or instrument that appears in published form. In all cases, the evaluator should contact the author and publisher to obtain permission to use the materials. In many cases, a letter of request is all that is needed, and permission will be granted for free. In other cases, though, the evaluator may need to purchase the rights to use the material. It is important for the evaluator to follow the appropriate procedures because such actions reflect on the evaluator as well as the organization.

5. Demonstrate awareness of the politics of evaluation. This competency includes the following three performance standards:

a) Identify the potential political implications of each evaluation.

b) Clarify stakeholder values.

c) Attend to political issues as they arise.

Twenty years ago, Carol Weiss (1987) introduced the importance of politics and values within any evaluation. When practitioners in the training or HR field are first asked to undertake an evaluation, they seldom think of it as a political activity. In fact, most evaluations are political *unless* they meet the criteria outlined by Michael Patton (1997, p. 352):

- No one cares about the program.

- No one knows about the program.

- No money is at stake.

- No power or authority is at stake.

If these criteria exist in a given situation, it is probably questionable as to whether the evaluation should even commence.

Evaluation by its very nature is political, and especially so when it feeds into a decision-making process. There are vested interests behind every program, process, or product that is evaluated. Often those charged with doing evaluation are at low levels in the organization and are faced with a conflict between laying out the facts or putting some sort of "spin" on the reporting.

Following are some examples of the kinds of political pressures that emerge in the course of an evaluation:

■ An evaluator is asked to evaluate the program championed by and introduced at the request of the CEO, but the data suggest that the program does not yield much value. The temptation would be to sanitize the findings or downplay the negatives.

■ An evaluator is given a list of people to interview, but they all seem to have the same bias (positive or negative) toward the program or delivery mode. The evaluator, then, wonders whether the interview data represent the true state of affairs or the views of a carefully chosen set of interviewees.

■ The evaluator suspects a stakeholder who receives a draft report will edit it to show more acceptable findings before it goes to the vice president.

■ The evaluator is asked to use a Likert-type survey with only four points on it to assess customer satisfaction, knowing that the smaller scale is biased toward a positive result.

One important strategy for managing the politics that may arise in an evaluation involves clarifying stakeholder values at the beginning of the evaluator process and reclarifying those throughout the process. Certainly, as part of the negotiation of a contract or evaluation plan, the evaluation should outline activities and responsibilities; an important aspect is to determine stakeholder involvement in the analysis and writing of the report. Included in such discussions would be the strategy of asking stakeholders to consider their reactions to alternative, possible findings.

Russ-Eft and Preskill (2001) provide some suggestions for managing the politics throughout the evaluation process. The following questions should be considered when assessing the potential political issues in an evaluation and determining appropriate actions:

■ Who championed the intervention?

■ Who has a vested interest in it continuing?

- Which stakeholders should be involved?

- How do I balance negative findings against positive ones?

- Who would stand to gain or lose if findings are used to make decisions or changes?

- How much credibility do I have?

PLANNING AND DESIGNING THE EVALUATION

The second competency domain is that of *Planning and Designing the Evaluation,* and it includes four competency areas:

- Evaluation planning

- Evaluation management planning

- Data collection strategies

- Pilot testing

The field of evaluation is characterized by an array of models, approaches, strategies, and frameworks. Despite their theoretical and practical differences, core among them is an emphasis on systematic conduct, a clear purpose (i.e., to improve program outcomes or effectiveness), and substantive outcomes that allow for generalizing the results and making recommendations. Evaluation is not merely about completing activities. As Patton (1997) states, evaluation is "the systematic collection of information about the activities, characteristics, and outcomes of programs to make judgments about the program, improve program effectiveness, and/ or inform decisions about future programming" (p. 23).

Practically speaking, then, the successful evaluation is based on a plan that is thoughtfully designed: comprehensive, methodologically robust, and flexible enough to be implemented and adapted as circumstances warrant. The following sections describe the competencies and performance statements associated with evaluation planning.

6. *Develop an effective evaluation plan.* This competency includes the following seven performance standards:

a) Describe the program, process, or product to be evaluated.

b) Identify the stakeholders.

c) Identify the evaluation focus and key questions to be answered.

d) Use best practices or relevant literature to guide the evaluation plan.

e) Describe the evaluation strategy and expected outcomes.

f) Identify models, methods, or designs to support the evaluation.

g) Collaborate with stakeholders to confirm the selected approach and evaluation design.

The evaluator must begin evaluation planning with a clear understanding of the evaluation program, process, or product and the context in which it operates. Basic fact finding is critical here, and this may help to reduce or eliminate political and other sorts of turmoil later in the evaluation. Review of program documents, semistructured interviews with program personnel, and informal observations of everyday operations help to reveal how the organization and the targeted program or process operate and are managed, who is involved and where they are located, and any relevant cultural factors. The evaluator needs to be very clear about exactly what is to be evaluated before moving further into the planning.

Also important early in the planning process is the identification of the key stakeholders. Stakeholders are individuals and groups who are involved in or affected by the performance and results of what is being evaluated. Like their business counterparts, evaluation stakeholders are defined as those with a vested interest in the program, process, or product being evaluated—and able to take advantage of the results.

Stakeholders can be differentiated by their level of investment and stake in the program. They include those who may have commissioned the evaluation or those with the authority to make operational decisions; these stakeholders plan to make instrumental use of the evaluation findings. In contrast, others have an interest in understanding program elements for planning purposes. Such stakeholders plan to make conceptual use of the evaluation.

In the case of a corporate training program, for example, stakeholders could include sponsors or champions of the program, the head of the company's training organization, instructional designers, instructors or facilitators, and participants and their managers. In organizations, the most often named stakeholder group tends to be employees or program participants. The most important group, however, may be the internal "customers," such as senior management, who will decide whether or not to continue supporting a program being evaluated. Sometimes stakeholder groups are unintentionally overlooked or deliberately ignored for political reasons. They could include community groups who will be affected by the outcome of a nonprofit agency evaluation, for example. In identifying the stakeholders, it is good practice to think in terms of concentric circles, beginning with the key stakeholder (usually the individual or group funding the program, requesting the evaluation, or both) and circling out to consider other groups or individuals who may have a vested interest in the evaluation process or outcomes. At the same time, the evaluator must begin to determine who among these stakeholders should have input in the evaluation and to what degree. Managing stakeholders, especially in a complex or large evaluation, is a critical skill area.

An evaluator must be able to identify who the stakeholders are and which of them should provide input to the evaluation study. Where there are political issues involved (e.g., the program was introduced by a senior executive who is very resistant to any suggested changes to it), the evaluator must be able to work with, involve, and incorporate input from key stakeholders without compromising the evaluation in any way. Important to note, however, is that evaluators—even when internal—face an array of constraints (e.g., tight budget, limited resources, short time line for data gathering, or limited access to data) that can compromise stakeholder identification and ongoing engagement.

As part of the evaluation plan, the evaluator must determine whether the evaluation is formative, summative, or both. A formative evaluation is improvement oriented; the focus is on what, if anything, needs to be revised or modified. The summative evaluation is more judgment oriented, responding to stakeholders who must determine whether or not or in what ways a program, process, or product has been effective, added value, accomplished its objectives, or met its goals. Minor changes may result from the evaluation effort, but improvement is *not* the primary outcome. Generally a summative evaluation is done only on a program that has been in place for some time, rather than after its first delivery. A summative evaluation of a new program can yield results showing a lack of success, simply because the program is still evolving.

The evaluator needs to be clear about the overriding goal or focus of the evaluation. It may help to consider the following:

- Do I have to find out what is working and what is not working and how to fix it?

- Do I have to find out how much participants are using what they have learned from this program?

- Do my stakeholders want to know if the program is adding value to our organization?

- Does this evaluation incorporate several of these issues?

Once the evaluator is clear about the overriding goal, a list of possible evaluation questions can be generated for review and discussion with the stakeholders. For each key question, the evaluator needs to be able to answer two questions: Why do we want to know this? And what will we do with the data? If the data will not be used, there is no point in collecting them. The final list of key questions will guide the design of the evaluation and, in particular, will suggest the data collection tools and where the data can be sourced.

Novice evaluators will find considerable assistance in planning this stage of the evaluation from one or two basic textbooks on evaluation (e.g., Russ-Eft & Preskill, 2001). These will provide insight on a variety of planning issues as well as on methods and tools to conduct the evaluation, given the key questions that have to be answered.

A hypothetical example helps to bring evaluation planning to life. Jones Enterprises is a midsized engineering and design firm. Executives are concerned about the development of first-line supervisors and have invested in a supervisory training program. Following are three approaches to planning an evaluation of this training; each illustrates the tension and interplay between and among three key tenets of planning design: *focus, strategy,* and *methods.*

With a *behavioral objectives* approach (as characterized in the work of Bloom, Engelhart, Furst, Hill, & Krathwohl, 1956; Mager, 1962; and Tyler, 1935), the evaluator begins by reviewing the specific goals and performance objectives of the training. The evaluator might want to know whether and how the goals and objectives are measured (such as ability to resolve conflict more effectively), whether they have been reviewed for relevancy, and how they align with the objectives of any other supervisory training programs at Jones Enterprises. Such an objectives-based evaluation will consider whether the objectives stated to be the basis of the program are in fact being met. Are supervisors now able to facilitate effective and productive team meetings? Do their staff members report an increase in the amount of communication and feedback?

A *management* approach would allow the evaluator to take a closer look at inputs, processes, and outputs (similar to the Input, Process, Output model by Bushnell [1990] or the CIPP approach by Stufflebeam [1983, 2000] described in Chapter 1). For example, the evaluator may want to examine the level of resources being allocated to the program, such as the quality of the training and instruction or the amount of time in training. Then the evaluator could identify the processes planned and accomplished for the program. These include such things as the learning management system: Is it manually tracked, or is there a computer-based system in place? It may include the selection of participants: How are people identified as potential attendees and notified that they will attend? Another process issue may involve monitoring: Is there a review process in place to monitor end-of-course evaluations and recommend changes to the design team? Finally, the evaluator could determine some of the outputs of the program. Such outputs could include measures of learning, such as test scores. Other outputs might focus on the behaviors of the attendees. To what extent are these supervisors better able to facilitate team meetings and deal with conflicts? Do managers report improved productivity among participating supervisors?

A *consumer* approach would allow the evaluator to focus on the constituents most involved in and affected by the training: the participants. Using this approach to the evaluation of Jones Enterprises supervisory training program, the evaluator might explore the experiences of the participants during training, their perceptions of its usefulness, and the extent to which they perceive their managers are supportive of the new skills they have learned.

While some specific framework or approach suggests a direction for the evaluation, in practical terms there is no one correct model or method. The major concern should be to provide useful and accurate data that answer the evaluation questions raised by the stakeholders and on which decision makers can act in relation to the program.

Although a review of the literature may seem unnecessary for busy professionals, it can lead to some cost and time savings. Through such a review, evaluators can gain some awareness of similar studies and some possible approaches. A good place to begin is with journal articles published by professional associations. In many cases, articles and conference papers are also available for downloading from association web sites. Refer to the list of professional associations and their web sites in Appendix E. Books are another source of information. The bibliography in Appendix D provides a list of basic evaluation books that are helpful in planning an evaluation. Finally, searching the Internet is an effective and rapid way of accessing information about all aspects of planning and conducting an evaluation.

When faced with planning an evaluation that is different from or more complex than those previously undertaken, an evaluator should also identify best practices for guidance. Often this is done through personal networks, which are good ways to identify best practices in other organizations, access information about how an evaluation was conducted, and possibly locate evaluation tools that can be adapted. Most large companies also subscribe to service organizations that provide members with relevant contacts in other companies, research reports on best practices, or information on how other companies have handled the same or a similar issue. Given the time constraints under which most evaluators work, it is important to be able to access information from the literature or other practitioners, rather than "reinventing the wheel" when planning an evaluation.

Engaging with stakeholders as part of the evaluation planning improves the quality of the effort by focusing its scope. Collaborating with stakeholders early in the evaluation planning process can aid in the selection and confirmation of the approach and the design. In addition, such early engagement can also boost stakeholders' receptivity to the recommendations or final report, even when the findings point to weaknesses that need to be addressed.

7. *Develop a management plan for the evaluation.* This competency includes the following nine performance statements:

   a) Develop the evaluation schedule, responsibilities, and deliverables.

   b) Determine the budget.

   c) Identify internal and external personnel requirements.

   d) Determine training needs of personnel.

   e) Determine technology requirements.

   f) Allocate personnel and resources to support the plan.

   g) Develop a communication and reporting plan.

   h) Obtain needed permissions regarding confidentiality.

   i) Prepare and negotiate a proposal.

Like a set of blueprints for a home construction or remodeling project, the management plan outlines the overall evaluation design, thereby ensuring sufficient resources to carry out the anticipated evaluation activities.

All evaluations need a management plan, even a routine evaluation of a regularly run program. The management plan should focus on the key questions and include a listing of the tasks, the expected time line to complete them, the technological resources required at each point, and the personnel needed if others are to be involved.

A budget with estimated costs should also be included where this is appropriate. Project costs may be both direct and indirect. Direct costs include staff salary and benefits (which often consume the largest portion of the budget), although for internal evaluations these are generally not factored into the evaluation budget. Other overt costs that an evaluator may have to take into account include consultants' fees and expenses, survey software if internal software and hosting are not available, communications, printing and duplication (if printed reports are required), data processing, copyright, supplies and equipment, and subcontracts (test development, data analysis, legal services, etc.). In some organizations, the evaluation may also need to include indirect costs. Such costs include office space and organizational services. Although developing a budget for each evaluation can be helpful, not all internal evaluations, particularly if they are done on a recurring basis, will require preparation of a budget.

Evaluators have several tools at their disposal for estimating the time and personnel requirements associated with task completion. The tools used will depend on the complexity of the evaluation and may include project management software such as Microsoft Excel, Microsoft Project, or Gantt charts, PERT charts, and the like. At a glance, then, the chart helps estimate when tasks should begin, what level of personnel effort may be needed, and anticipated task duration; and its use helps gauge progress to date of the evaluation. The simplicity and straightforward nature of Gantt charts make them useful to share with key stakeholders also.

An evaluator plays many roles as manager—from supervising the evaluation team to serving as a liaison to stakeholders and participants in the evaluation. The manager oversees the project and, where necessary, must mediate conflicts, address concerns others raise, and solve problems raised during the evaluation process.

Large-scale evaluations generally involve more than one person. The effort will fail or be seriously compromised if staff members are not fully qualified to carry out the evaluation tasks. In choosing evaluation team members, the evaluator must consider both the skills required and the workload. The evaluation may require external consultants, such as coordinators, data gatherers, or data analysts, if internal personnel lack these skill sets or are unavailable. Evaluation is an opportunity for collaboration between and among different divisions, sectors, or departments, even within a small organization. The internal evaluator can strengthen relationships (and perhaps reduce the anxiety that evaluation often produces) by involving different groups in the effort.

Sometimes an evaluator determines that factors other than technical skills are important in selecting staff for the project. Let's return to Jones Enterprises. A key task in the evaluation is to interview people who, within the past three months, have received training in diversity and cultural awareness. The evaluator has two staff members from which to choose: one with strong interviewing skills, the other lacking those skills but whose own background, personal experiences, and interpersonal skills make that person very credible to the target group. In this case, the evaluator makes a selection based on interpersonal skills and credibility rather than technical skills and provides training to enhance overall readiness to perform.

The evaluator may be forced to work with personnel with little or no prior experience in evaluation. The cost and time needed for training such staff must be determined. Even staff members with relevant expertise require basic orientation to the evaluation project and how it will unfold. Obviously, those needs increase when staff members are inexperienced or lack familiarity with or exposure to the setting, context, specific tasks, or target groups. Knowing the strengths and weaknesses of each team member helps the evaluator tailor the training offered. The focus, for example, might be cultural, technological, procedural, technical, or even ethical. The evaluator must build supervision time into the management plan, which may involve reviewing an individual's work or checking that person's knowledge and skills for the various tasks being undertaken.

Although monitoring the management plan is discussed elsewhere in this chapter, it is important to note here that the plan depicts the way evaluation oversight or monitoring will unfold. A calendar-oriented management plan (where activities are spelled out by date) calls for monitoring on a fairly predictable schedule, such as each week, every other week, or each month. Most project management specialists advocate for a plan organized around milestones associated with the specified tasks. This enables the evaluator to keep the key deliverables in focus and make changes or adapt to unanticipated issues in a timely manner. A management plan based on milestones enables the evaluator to recognize problems, as they begin to emerge, that will impact the time frame, the budget, or both, and to take proactive steps to minimize the problem.

Designing the management plan is best undertaken as a collaborative activity, with the evaluator consulting key stakeholders as it is developed; this proactive stance ensures that the evaluator and key stakeholders work together. Such collaboration is more likely to bring to the surface issues that might compromise the effort; for example, difficulties with data collection efforts or possible staff changes. Based on discussions with stakeholders, the evaluator might opt to modify the evaluation—for example, by narrowing its scope, redesigning the data collection plan to use existing measures, or replacing a labor-intensive technique with one easier and less costly to implement.

Developing a communication and reporting plan is one step that is critical to ensuring use of the evaluation findings. First, it is important to think of the communication and reporting as consisting of more than just the final report. Keeping stakeholders informed of progress can help to ensure continued cooperation and support. Furthermore, there is sometimes a need for interim reports, and it is helpful for the evaluator to know about and plan for such reports. When functioning as an external consultant, the evaluator will need to prepare a draft report. In some instances, this is presented in an oral and written manner to the primary internal contact or the executive team. That report and presentation will then be reviewed, and input will be given for revisions before finalizing it. Working on the scheduling of reports is one issue, but the effective evaluator also considers the format of the report. In most cases, the culture of the organization will dictate whether the report should be text based or should simply consist of a PowerPoint presentation. In a military organization, the report generally needs to be in numbered paragraphs. Attention to the scheduling and the format of reports contributes a great deal to the eventual acceptance of the findings and recommendations for action.

Unlike a research study, an evaluation is undertaken in order to lead to some action. Such action can occur only if the findings and recommendations are communicated to the key people. It is therefore advisable to involve stakeholders in the review and interpretation of the findings and to plan for this involvement from the start. When the evaluator is an external consultant, such involvement becomes even more important because the stakeholders may recognize the organizational significance of certain findings not noticed by the consultant. The evaluator must recognize, however, that there are some inherent dangers in this level of stakeholder involvement. What if some stakeholders do not like what they read in the interim report? Back at Jones Enterprises, the sales director's newly introduced sales skills training has not been rated very highly, and an early analysis of sales data seems to confirm the program's ineffectiveness. The evaluator knows the sales director is not going to be enthusiastic about abandoning a program that he has advocated throughout his division.

The section on competency 4 above, dealing with ethical and legal standards, introduced some ideas concerning confidentiality and anonymity. Although an evaluator may possess knowledge of such standards, it is important to inform the client and stakeholders of the need for confidentiality and anonymity throughout the data collection and analysis. As part of this sharing, the effective evaluator will craft appropriate statements concerning confidentiality and anonymity and will share these with the client and stakeholders. Furthermore, the needed permissions must be obtained throughout the process.

A final issue for the evaluator involves the development and negotiation of a formal proposal for the evaluation. If working as an external evaluator, the need for a proposal may be obvious. An internal evaluator will, however, be well served by preparing and negotiating such a proposal. The proposal should contain (1) a brief description of the program, process, or product; (2) the stakeholders and their involvement; (3) the evaluation focus and key questions; (4) the model, methods, or designs supporting the evaluation; (5) the evaluation schedule, responsibilities, and deliverables; (6) the communication and reporting plan; (7) the budget and other needed resources, including technology; and (8) internal and external personnel requirements and their training needs. By outlining these areas, the evaluator has provided the client and the stakeholder with information as to what they can expect from and about the evaluation effort.

8. *Devise data collection strategies to support the evaluation questions and design.* This competency includes the following nine performance statements:

a) Identify potential data sources.

b) Draw on a variety of evaluation instruments and procedures.

c) Evaluate the appropriateness of using existing instruments and tools.

d) Construct reliable and valid instruments.

e) Develop a data collection plan, including protocols and procedures.

f) Design appropriate sampling procedures.

g) Address threats to trustworthiness and validity of data.

h) Develop a plan for data analysis and interpretation.

i) Plan for the storage, security, and disposal of data.

This competency lies at the heart of an evaluation. Possessing strong foundational skills; collaborating with stakeholders; building a budget and evaluation plan; and identifying needed staff, consultants, or both lay the groundwork for what may be considered the critical components of an evaluation.

Evaluators have various ways to document the data collection strategy. A common approach is to create a template that can be adapted to fit each evaluation. Such a template is in the form of a matrix listing the key questions, the type of information required to answer each question, the potential sources for that information, and the best methods to capture the information (e.g., survey, interview, review and analysis of documents).

Although the evaluator factors in the budget, time frame, and an array of logistical issues to decisions about data sources, it is wise to begin with a big-picture approach and consider all the possibilities where data might be found. A first choice might be existing data; reports, performance management reviews and other HR documentation, memos, specifications and test plans, meeting agenda and minutes, policies and guidelines, and work products are examples of where one might find data addressing the evaluation questions. Generally the data are internal to the organization, but in some cases they may be external or public, readily available in print or electronically. Such organizational artifacts often provide rich sources of information for evaluators to use.

Because people are at the heart of most programs or processes that evaluators examine, they are a primary data source. Among the many firsthand information sources on which an evaluator may draw are program participants; instructors or facilitators; and those who interact with participants, such as supervisors, coworkers, subordinates, and customers. In some cases, evaluators are interested in data that they cannot draw directly from people connected with a program. For example, the organization is interested in the effectiveness of a customer service program but is not willing for the evaluator to have any contact with customers. In such a case, the evaluator must find indirect ways to assess customer perceptions. Sometimes the evaluator can use customer satisfaction reports that have been collected from within the company by another department or done by an external organization. From these, the evaluator can draw out relevant data to support or add to findings from his or her own data collection.

Access to data is an issue that many evaluators face. Sometimes the data they need simply are not available to them; other times there is a subtle opposition to the collection of such information. For example, organizational policies may preclude employees from speaking openly because their comments involve highly sensitive proprietary information. Or the corporate culture may not encourage those selected for interviews to be candid if their comments can be construed as negative in some way. The evaluator may not be able to assure anonymity or confidentiality. Stakeholders, particularly if they hold a powerful position within the organization, may exert pressure on the evaluator to *not* ask certain questions. The evaluator will have to consider how much the final report should document the constraints to data gathering.

In determining what instruments to use, evaluators must first ask, Who provides the information? There are three primary categories. The first category is extant, or existing, data or records, which the evaluator will request permission to examine. For example, the evaluator could review the content of a training manual to determine how closely it aligns with the performance objectives. Or the evaluator could examine performance management reports to determine how well managers are writing performance goals for each person who reports to them. A second category is the recipients of the program, process, or product being evaluated. Typically these are course participants or product or process users. They may be directly involved (course participants, users of a process or product) or indirectly involved (managers or employees who report directly to the participants). The third category is knowledgeable others. For example, in evaluating the success of an organizational change initiative, knowledgeable others could include organizational development personnel who developed and deployed the initiative. What is important, however, is to take the time to think about the different categories of data source in relation to the evaluation questions. Too often training evaluations rely on surveys of course participants and fail to consider which other sources could provide useful information.

Data may be collected using various methods including surveys, tests, performance assessments, 360-feedback reports, interviews, focus groups, observations, and review of existing documents and participant action plans. The choice of the particular method or methods will depend on the goals of the evaluation as well as project constraints, particularly budget and time. For example, an evaluator assessing the effectiveness of a new procedure for factory supervisors may feel that three or four focus groups of supervisors would be the best data collection method. Unfortunately, the evaluator does not have sufficient time to run all of these focus groups, or alternatively, the supervisors cannot get permission to leave the factory floor for the 30 minutes needed.

Survey forms generally consist of scaled, multiple-choice, check-all-that-apply, or dichotomous items, making the data gathered mostly quantitative in nature. Many times, however, surveys also have open-ended questions that allow respondents to provide qualitative data. Surveys are well suited for situations where data will be gathered from large numbers, especially if respondents are geographically dispersed. Protocol forms for individual interviews and focus groups can capture both qualitative and quantitative data. Observation forms, too, may be designed to gather qualitative data (e.g., assessing performance against a checklist) or quantitative data (e.g., observing performance in an interpersonal interaction and assessing its effectiveness). In this case, the evaluator may observe directly or use media to capture the original information for later review.

Creating valid and reliable evaluation tools is time-consuming and difficult. An important consideration is the disciplinary or domain expertise that the design and development of an instrument demands. Reliability and validity must be addressed, even when fashioned with experts and carefully pilot tested. When it is feasible to do so, an evaluator will want to repurpose existing tools. This is often possible with surveys and interview protocols that can be adapted. For more complex or large-scale evaluations, the evaluator may opt to use standardized tools that professionals have prepared and thoroughly tested. A number of databases are useful tool sources as well, including *Tests in Print* (Buros Institute, 2006), *Buros Mental Measurement Yearbook* (Buros Institute, 2007), WilsonWeb (http://hwwilsonweb.com), EBSCO (http://www.ebsco.com), ProQuest (http://proquest.com), and Google Scholar (http://scholar.google.com). With permission, an evaluator may be able to adapt an existing instrument to meet a project's unique needs without compromising the tool's integrity.

Because evaluations can be tainted by instruments that lack scientific rigor, evaluators must deal with the issues of reliability and validity.

Validity is the degree to which the items or the instrument measure what they are intended to measure. Reliability refers to the degree or level of measurement error that exists in the data collection tool or in the actual data. Thus, an instrument or data considered to be reliable would have little or no error, leading to consistency in the measurement from one administration of the instrument to the next. In other words, if an evaluator administers the instrument (considered reliable) to the participants on two occasions, the results will be similar (or even identical). Unfortunately, an instrument can be reliable but not valid; in other words, it can yield comparable responses from the same group of people if administered on more than one occasion, but it does not accurately represent the concept being measured. In a common example, patients can consistently weigh themselves on their home scales, but the results may not agree with those from a calibrated scale in a physician's office. An example in an organizational context might involve the use of a survey that consistently shows positive results from training, but such results do not appear when using a validated instrument. Clearly, this is a serious problem!

The Joint Committee on Educational and Psychological Tests (1999) produced the most recent statement on test and instrument validity, *Standards for Educational and Psychological Testing*. It described six types of validity. First, "face validity" simply indicates that a casual review confirms the instrument appears to be measuring what it claims to measure. Second, "validity based on test content" refers to a more thorough and detailed examination of the content and format of the instrument (whether it truly represents the concepts of interest). This type of validity tends to come from the review of experts or those with some expertise in that particular domain. Third, "validity based on response processes" involves an examination of the responses to determine whether the instrument measures what it claims to measure. Fourth, "validity based on internal structure" uses statistical analyses to confirm the factor structure of the instrument as another indication that it is measuring what it purports to measure. Fifth, "validity based on relations to other variables" uses statistical analyses to compare the instruments with other related instruments and variables. Sixth, "validity based on consequences" examines the consequences of the instrument to ensure that it measures what it claims to measure. These various concepts replace and subsume the earlier notions of face, content, criterion, predictive, and construct validity.

Another consideration involves threats to the trustworthiness and validity of the instrument and the resulting data. Poor question wording and instrument design represent some of the most frequent threats. A common error is to ask about two separate issues in one question, for example, *How would you rate the design and execution of the seminar?* Another typical error involves the use of scaled responses that are skewed to give a favorable response. This can be seen in customer satisfaction surveys that have a multiple-point scale in which most of the points are favorable. Simply based on the scale, one could predict an 85 percent satisfaction rating. If the survey is not anonymous, asking for opinions that are likely to be negative can also create problems because respondents may be unwilling to say what they really think. Also, faulty interpretation and misuse of the data can yield results that are invalid.

Sampling is another potential threat to validity. Incorrect sampling or too small a sample are common mistakes made by novice evaluators. Furthermore, sampling must be considered in any study. With small-scale studies where the number of potential participants (or documents or artifacts to examine) is already limited, the evaluator may decide to involve the entire population. For instance, if only 25 people have attended the training program, it would be wise to use all of them in the evaluation. In evaluations that are largely qualitative in nature, the evaluator can choose among a menu of options:

■ *Purposive*: The evaluator establishes criteria to chose a small number of cases that fairly and accurately represent all the main issues, questions, or positions.

■ *Convenience*: Select a sample of the population or information sources that are easily accessible.

■ *Snowball*: The evaluator might contact departments within an organization and ask for suggestions about potential information sources, and those sources provide additional leads or ideas.

An evaluator whose approach is more quantitative in nature or involves many people and information sources may opt instead for more rigorous sampling methods, such as randomly selecting participants (or other information sources) from the larger population. Such random sampling can occur with the entire group (considered a simple random sample) or in proportions that represent specific groups (considered a stratified random sample). Such stratification may be important when there are concerns about including people from specific groups, particularly if a particular group contains a small number of people. If the evaluation requires such sampling procedures, it may be wise to hire a statistical expert to help at this stage of the evaluation plan. Many textbooks (e.g., Russ-Eft & Preskill, 2001) provide charts to help determine the number of people to be sampled. One can also use an online calculator, such as http://www.surveysystem .com/sscalc.htm.

Considerable work precedes data analysis (e.g., organizing, sorting, coding). A data analysis or interpretive plan provides the road map an evaluator follows to determine how the various data elements fit together to address the evaluation questions. For example, in evaluating a program to train managers to mentor others, the evaluator might combine survey data about mentees' perceptions, observations of the training, and interviews with mentors to provide a composite view of program effectiveness.

In the data analysis section of the plan, the evaluator describes the statistical or summarizing techniques to be employed for analyzing the information and how these activities will be undertaken. The section of the plan dealing with data interpretation, on the other hand, informs decisions the evaluator makes about the format or structure of the analysis for reporting purposes. Decisions about interpretation help to determine where graphic support (tables, graphs, charts, or figures) or direct quotes (if individuals cannot be personally identified by their inclusion) will be used to improve reader understanding of the findings. Attention to both analysis and interpretation helps the evaluator prepare a report that assists key stakeholders make next-step decisions.

Planning for the storage, security, and disposal of the data should also be considered when developing the data collection strategy. Throughout the project, the evaluator must determine how the data will be handled, by whom, and in what manner. By implication, then, the evaluator must continually be in control of the data; data cannot be made available to those who might deliberately or inadvertently cause harm. Specifically, the evaluator must clarify with the stakeholders that the data represent sensitive information and are "owned" by the evaluator. Therefore, data should always be stored in a secure location to which only the evaluator has access so that confidentiality is maintained. At the conclusion of the project, typically about six months after delivering the final report, the evaluator should destroy all records, particularly those that contain confidential information. Such records include not only written documents but also any audiotapes or videotapes of interviews or focus groups.

9. *Pilot test the data collection instruments and procedures.* This competency includes the following three performance statements:

a) Design the pilot test.

b) Identify an appropriate sample.

c) Implement changes based on feedback and results.

Instrument testing is a critical component of evaluation planning. No matter how carefully the tools are developed, pilot testing ensures the instruments are reliable and valid, appropriate for the target group, and aligned with the evaluation questions and focus.

An evaluator may employ one of several testing strategies. When the instruments target specific types of respondents, the evaluator most often turns to purposive sampling to select members of the target audience for the testing; they complete the survey or are interviewed using the agreed-on protocols, and they are asked to provide feedback about the clarity, comprehensiveness, length, time to complete, and language appropriateness. Researcher-developed instruments are often tested by peers or, more likely, experts in the targeted domain or discipline. Whereas each provides a different perspective, together they can pinpoint potential threats to validity and reliability.

Pilot testing is best conducted in the environment or setting in which actual data collection will take place, although that is not always possible. A common error is the failure to account for delivery or implementation differences. For example, if a survey is to be web-based, the pilot test should not use a paper-based version. In addition, with web-based surveys, the pilot test is an opportunity to ensure that the data collection software is capturing all the data. This is particularly important when the software is linked to internal demographic information that will be pulled across into the data collection. Pilot testing will reveal whether or not this is actually occurring as planned.

Pilot testing of instruments is not done as often as it should be in the corporate environment. This may be because the evaluator is under pressure to begin data collection as soon as possible or simply does not realize the purpose of pilot testing. Nevertheless, pilot testing can help to ensure that survey questions are clear and unambiguous, that all online survey data are being captured by the system, including demographic data, and finally, that survey forms and interview or focus group protocols are generating data that address the evaluation questions. Pilot testing, then, represents some quality assurance and will reduce the likelihood of problems during data collection.

The evaluator should, however, never take the actual results of the pilot test too seriously, given the small sample and the lack of statistical power. The effort is really about making adjustments to problems with the data collection process and instruments. It should not be used as a substitute for the full evaluation effort.

IMPLEMENTING THE EVALUATION PLAN

The third competency domain is that of *Implementing the Evaluation Plan,* and it includes three competency areas:

- Data collection

- Data analysis and interpretation

- Dissemination

The previous domain, *Planning and Designing the Evaluation,* relates to the development of the plan, budget, and schedule for the evaluation. This domain involves the actual conduct of this plan. Although excellent execution of these competencies cannot guarantee an effective and successful evaluation, faulty or incomplete data collection, analysis, and dissemination will result in inaccuracies, misinterpretation, and misuse or nonuse of the evaluation. The following paragraphs describe each of the competencies and their associated performance statements along with some discussion of the competency.

10.   Collect data. The seven performance statements detailing this competency are as follows:

   a) Implement the data collection plan, schedule, and budget.

   b) Document evaluation activities.

   c) Conduct effective individual or group interviews.

   d) Conduct effective observations.

   e) Record and summarize relevant existing data.

   f) Respond to changes in the scope or focus of the evaluation.

   g) Minimize disruptions during data collection.

Data collection begins once the evaluation plan is in place and is the heart of the implementation phase. The evaluator follows the data collection plan, working within the allotted budget and time schedule as much as possible. However, during the data collection, unanticipated problems can emerge, posing difficulties in both cost and time lines. For example, scheduling interviews becomes problematic because of a company crisis that requires the attention of many of the prospective interviewees. Or in the case of a web-based survey, there is a technical or software problem that did not show up in the pilot testing. Experienced evaluators build in additional time and budget, especially in large evaluations, to cover for these contingencies.

It is critical that all data collection activities are thoroughly documented. It is wise to systematically document each step of the data collection, along with the related findings. As well as the results of the data collection, the documentation should include such information as the date(s) when the data were gathered, the location(s) of the data collection, the individuals who participated, and the people who collected the data. The evaluator should also record any unusual events or responses that occurred during the data collection. For example, any special organizational announcements, such as mergers or layoffs, should be noted. To the extent possible, documenting is a task to be done at the time of the data collection because delays in documentation can result in important information being lost or forgotten. Because most evaluations gather information that should remain confidential, this documentation should be maintained in a secure location.

As noted earlier, there are many methods for collecting data. Those most commonly used in organizations are surveys, questionnaires, interviews, focus groups, observations, and reviews of documents and artifacts. Other possibilities include tests and simulations. Although most evaluators tend to have preferred methods, perhaps because of the type of evaluation they most often undertake, it is recommended that they be familiar with and competent in each of these data collection methods. Competence involves understanding not only the procedures used in each method but also the advantages and disadvantages and the most appropriate data collection setting for the various methods.

When considering the use of interviews, several decisions must be made. First, the evaluator must decide whether to undertake individual interviews or conduct focus groups. Individual interviews can be conducted in person or by phone and allow for personal perspectives of the interviewees to emerge. A disadvantage may be the amount of time to complete them. In contrast, focus groups enable the evaluator to collect data from a number of people when time is of the essence. Some disadvantages are that strong opinions may predominate and it is more difficult to pursue a line of questioning based on one person's experience or views. Because there can be a lot of cross-group dialogue, the evaluator usually focuses on facilitating the group and has an assistant take notes.

When conducting interviews, whether individual or group, the evaluator needs to think about how to make the interviewees feel emotionally comfortable. One important aspect influencing that comfort level as well as reducing the intrusiveness and disruption to others in the organization, is the interview location. Whenever possible, an interview should be held in a private room or office. If this is not possible, sitting in the far corner of the company cafeteria or moving to an outside location can be considered. The evaluator should ensure that the participants receive written information about the purpose, the location, and the timing of the interview. At the beginning of the interview, it is good practice to reiterate the purpose and importance of the interview, indicate how it relates to the overall evaluation, describe what will happen to the information that is shared, agree on the time allocated for it, and outline the procedures for maintaining confidentiality. The evaluator should ask the interviewees or focus groups questions as though this were a conversation. By moving away from a formal interview setting and approach to a more conversational one, the evaluator can often get much better qualitative data. During the interview, it is important to remain neutral but not passive; conveying interest in what is being said is different from agreeing with everything that is being said. This is particularly important when interview or focus group data are aligned with what the evaluator privately thinks about the program or process being evaluated. An aspect of professionalism is to remain neutral and listen for the opposite point of view.

The evaluator must also decide how to record the information being gathered in the interview or focus group. Taking notes on a laptop during the interview or focus group may result in some loss of important details and may cause the evaluator to appear distracted. On the other hand, using a tape recorder or video recorder will lead to additional time for transcription, and many interviewees are uncomfortable with their comments being permanently recorded on tape. Another related option involves using a digital recorder. Some analysis systems facilitate the uploading and coding of digital recordings, which can maintain authenticity and reduce error. (Such digital recordings do not necessarily reduce the amount of time for coding, however.) If the decision is made to tape or record interview or focus-group sessions, the evaluator must gain the interviewees' permission to do so as well as permission in writing from relevant stakeholders. Failure to do so could lead to a legal issue in some settings.

When considering doing group interviews, the evaluator should explore the use of technology such as audio- or videoconferencing.

Skype (http://www.skype.com) is also a good option when budgets are limited and interviewees (either singly or in small groups) are located in different parts of the world. In such cases, the evaluator should check the procedures for the conference call setup, making sure that participants have not only the correct call-in information but also alternate numbers if problems arise. Another alternative would be to set up online discussions for asynchronous or real-time interviewing. With real-time options, including Skype, the evaluator should be aware of the level of security provided.

In the right setting, observations provide another useful means for gathering data. These can document whether or not certain behaviors and procedures are being used on the job. Observing at intervals over a period of time tends to minimize the perceived intrusiveness as well as data collection burden. However, it does lengthen the data collection period. Observation is often done with the evaluator assessing performance in relation to a checklist of tasks. Such checklists or worksheets can help to ensure reliability among multiple observers, and simple procedures to ensure inter-rater reliability can be found in basic evaluation texts.

Evaluators sometimes overlook the fact that useful data matching the evaluation need may already exist in the organization. For example, needs assessments done before the development of a training program are usually informative about the existing skills of the target population, among other things. It may be possible to access performance management or 360-feedback data from the HR department when evaluating managers who have attended an advanced leadership program. An organization with an online mentoring program can run reports that reveal which groups of learners have signed on, how often they have engaged with their mentee, and how both mentor and mentee rate the relationship. Evaluators, especially external consultants who do not have intimate insider knowledge of the organization should always inquire about what data already exist that would shed light on the evaluation questions, and they should request access to relevant records, documents, and files. It is worthwhile to develop a template outlining the kinds of information needed and to document the records examined.

All data collection activities must be conducted so that they are unobtrusive and cause minimal disruption within the organization. Such intrusions and disruptions can occur with any data collection effort, but remaining unobtrusive is particularly important when observing employees performing their jobs. Observations enable the evaluator to view people within their work setting, but the presence of an observer may influence the activity being observed. It is, therefore, ideal for the observer to be in an inconspicuous location if possible. But employees may, in fact, be aware that observations are being conducted; thus, surreptitious observation may be impossible. On other occasions, data collection may require an evaluator to seek manager permission to have employees leave their work stations for a significant amount of time (e.g., a 30-minute interview). Such interviews need to be scheduled so as to reduce the impact on the workflow. With surveys and interviews, there may be particular times of the year when data collection will cause problems for the employees or the organization. For example, senior managers in large organizations are preoccupied with budgets and results data, particularly at the end of each fiscal quarter (or at year's end) and will not be available for interviews during such times. Even document reviews are best scheduled so that the review does not inconvenience employees who need access to the documents to complete their work. This may require the evaluator to do this review work before or after normal work hours.

Despite careful and thorough planning, an evaluator must be prepared for changes in the scope or focus of the evaluation as it progresses. These changes may ultimately lead to needed changes in the data collection effort, such as adding new data collection methods, changing the data collection methods, or increasing or decreasing the number of people to be interviewed. What is critical is to keep everyone involved in the evaluation informed of the changes and to make certain that the changes receive needed approval as well as any needed adjustments to the budget and schedule.

11. Analyze and interpret data. This competency includes the following five important performances:

a) Assess the trustworthiness, validity, and reliability of data.

b) Use appropriate quantitative or qualitative analysis procedures.

c) Review and interpret data in an unbiased way.

d) Make judgments about the findings and draw conclusions.

e) Develop recommendations.

Once data are collected, the evaluator will be keen to begin the analysis phase. Before moving into analysis, however, it is important to assess the trustworthiness of the data. In other words, can the data be trusted? Do the data represent the "truth" or the reality concerning the program, the process, or the product? Or does some bias exist in the data?

Trustworthiness applies to both quantitative and qualitative data. Certainly, one can examine the consistency of the data that have been gathered. If a team conducts observations or interviews or codes data for example, it is important that members adopt a consistent approach. An evaluator can do this through checking the inter-rater reliability, for example, or through a review of an audit trail on the data collection.

Several different methods exist for examining the trustworthiness of qualitative data. *Member checking* involves the interviewees in reviewing and confirming the data and the analyses. In this case, interview transcripts might be reviewed and confirmed with participants; alternatively, the themes emerging from the interviews might be reviewed and confirmed. *Data triangulation* involves undertaking a comparison among data from several different sources. Thus, the evaluator might gather perceptions of a particular program from supervisory participants, their managers, and those who report directly to them. Is there some alignment among the responses? In *method triangulation,* the evaluator compares data collected through different methods. For example, during analysis, the evaluator cross-checks the answers given on a survey question with the information shared in an interview asking a similar question. *Investigator triangulation* implies that several different researchers are involved in the data collection and analysis. *Peer debriefing* refers to involving a peer in reviewing and possibly interpreting or reinterpreting the results.

In deciding on the most appropriate analysis procedure, the evaluator will review the key questions for the evaluation as well as consider the expectations and knowledge of the stakeholders. Providing key stakeholders, who possess little background in statistics, with a comprehensive analysis based on sophisticated statistical techniques may not prove as useful as providing a number of carefully selected anecdotes from interviews. In contrast, presenting statistical analyses to stakeholders with an engineering background may aid in an understanding and appreciation of the results.

With quantitative data, the evaluator can begin by simply describing the data. Such data descriptions include frequency distributions, measures of central tendency (such as the mean, mode, and median), and perhaps, measures of variability (such as the standard deviation, interquartile range, and range), where it is important to understand how similar or different the responses are. There may be cases where the types of data that have been collected lend themselves to statistical analysis, which would provide insights not otherwise gained. In this case, evaluators need to employ the services of someone with expertise and background in statistical analyses if they lack this background themselves. For internal evaluators, there is usually such a person within the organization or an external consultant available on call to the organization.

Qualitative analyses, also called *content analyses* or *thematic analyses,* involve classifying the data or determining themes or patterns in the data. The evaluator might decide to code interview data, for example, according to the key questions driving the evaluation. Alternatively, the evaluator can allow the categories to emerge from the data by grouping similar comments from interviews or open-ended survey questions under headings and analyzing the themes that surface. In either case, the evaluator should keep clear and detailed records as to the procedures used, both for the purpose of establishing an audit trail and for member checking and peer debriefing.

In all cases, however, the evaluator needs to go beyond descriptive reporting. Novice evaluators tend to report the ratings for each question on a survey, list the open-ended comments without any kind of grouping, and then assume that the interpretation is self-evident. Evaluators need to sort through the data, organize them, look for patterns and themes, and provide an analysis. This represents their added value to the client and stakeholders.

An evaluator must take great care to review and interpret the resulting data and analyses in an unbiased way. This means being careful to control personal biases or views from influencing the analysis and summary of findings. For example, in the case of Jones Enterprises, the evaluator may personally believe that the program is poorly designed and much less effective than it should be for the cost involved. However, the data show that participants enjoyed the program, found it applicable to their jobs, and have applied much of what they learned. Furthermore, their managers are satisfied with the changes they see among attendees in the way they handle their teams. In this case, the evaluator needs to report the positive results and not allow personal negative views about the program to influence the recommendations.

The evaluator's job is to go beyond the analysis; the person must provide an interpretation of the results and recommendations for action based on the data. Recommendations need to be related to the evaluation focus and questions. But often insights that were not anticipated emerge from the evaluation and lead to a recommendation. For example, it becomes apparent that the participants in an effective meetings program who reported the greatest reduction in the amount of time spent on routine meetings were those who shared with their supervisor what they had learned and how they intended to use it. This then leads to a recommendation that at the end of this course, participants and supervisors should talk about how the principles learned in the effective meetings course are going to be implemented in all future departmental meetings.

One question that may arise is, *How does the evaluator decide when the data are pointing to a recommendation?* If, for example, 20 percent of the respondents indicate that a course was too long, should this be the basis for a recommendation that it be shortened? This is where triangulation is helpful. Specifically, are there results from other data sources or other data methods that point to the same conclusion and that would lead to this recommendation?

The evaluator needs to think through the consequences of each recommendation. This means considering the reactions of the various stakeholders, particularly in light of their values as suggested in competency 5 concerning the politics of evaluation. Furthermore, the evaluator should substantiate any recommendation and be able to provide the relevant data. For example, if the evaluator suggests that a training program be discontinued and a senior manager asks for "proof" that the data support that recommendation, the evaluator needs to be able to do so.

In developing these recommendations, it is helpful to involve stakeholders in reviewing the findings, assisting with their interpretation, and helping to craft the next-step actions. By involving stakeholders, the evaluator is more likely to ensure that the recommended actions are realistic and likely to be implemented.

12. Disseminate and follow up the findings and recommendations. This competency includes the following four performance guidelines:

 a) Use multiple methods of communicating and reporting.

 b) Discuss and interpret the evaluation findings with stakeholders.

 c) Present the findings according to the needs of diverse audiences.

 d) Facilitate or monitor changes resulting from recommendations.

An evaluation should lead to some decision-making and action. This can occur only if the evaluation and its recommendations are disseminated to stakeholders. As mentioned in previous sections, stakeholder involvement in the development of the recommendations helps with support, but it is only through some dissemination of the evaluation that wider acceptance can be achieved.

Communication and reporting need not take place only at the end of the evaluation. It is important to continuously inform stakeholders about the progress of the evaluation. Such communication can be undertaken in a variety of ways. The most common is a regular, brief but formal progress report to the key stakeholders, possibly each week. Usually this can be done by e-mail, but some organizations prefer a PowerPoint presentation at a departmental meeting, for example. Other communications may include short articles for the organization's newsletter or brief e-mails to selected individuals over the course of the evaluation if the study covers a longer period. Such communication helps to maintain interest in and support for the evaluation.

An effective evaluator can use the communication sessions with stakeholders to discuss and interpret the findings. Such sessions can prove beneficial in helping not only the stakeholders but also the evaluator to understand the findings and identify important recommendations.

At the conclusion of an evaluation, the evaluator prepares a final report in which are presented the findings and the recommendations. The format of this report should be given careful thought. Multiple approaches may be helpful where there are a large number of stakeholders. In most cases, executives will prefer a brief executive summary or a short presentation. In contrast, those involved in the development and implementation of the program will probably prefer more detailed information, both in writing and in some oral presentation or discussion.

Most organizations have preferences for reporting. For example, in one organization, the evaluator may be one of several people presenting various reports at a departmental meeting and be given 15 minutes to present half a dozen PowerPoint slides summing up the findings and recommendations. In another organization, the preferred way may be a detailed written report. In a third, the requirement may be for a two-page-maximum executive summary, which is all that the key decision makers will review. Failure to take organizational preferences into account may in some cases result in the report not being read.

For many evaluators, especially those who are external consultants, the presentation of the report happens at the end of the evaluation. They are not involved in the discussion of the findings or the implementation of the recommendations. Where it is possible to remain involved, the evaluator can work with the stakeholders and facilitate or monitor changes that result from the report. This is more likely to occur if the evaluator is an employee of the organization But even those who act as external evaluation consultants to the organization can continue to engage with the organization to facilitate use of the findings and recommendations.

MANAGING THE EVALUATION

The competency domain, *Managing the Evaluation,* focuses on the technical and dynamic aspects of evaluation project management. The competencies in this domain pertain to:

▪ Monitoring the evaluation plan

▪ Working effectively with personnel and stakeholders

13. Monitor the management plan. This competency includes the following five performance standards:

    a) Adapt the plan to meet changing circumstances.

    b) Review and adjust the budget, if needed.

    c) Track evaluation progress against schedule.

    d) Identify and resolve problems that arise during evaluation.

    e) Foster reflection and dialogue on the evaluation process and outcomes.

Project management is a general label for the techniques used in taking overall responsibility for the planning and managing of the activities needed to complete the evaluation on time and within budget. When an evaluator is not working alone on a project but has a team or various individuals assisting (e.g., an information technology [IT] specialist, an HR person, and a team member), the project management role becomes one of monitoring the progress of each person in terms of the overall milestones established in the evaluation plan.

Competent evaluators, especially those who work as a team leader, will assume that projects will not go according to plan and thus are constantly in need of monitoring. Their role involves tracking and adjusting progress, identifying and resolving problems, and communicating changes and impact to final products. They adjust project milestone dates, deliverables, and sometimes personnel to achieve the final product as necessary. A number of project management products can be used, such as Microsoft Project (http://office.microsoft.com/en-us/project/default.aspx), Daptiv (http://www.daptiv.com/), or Open Workbench (http://www.openworkbench.org), to create, monitor, and adjust evaluation project plans. These packages help to track and communicate progress and changes in tasks, responsibilities, and time lines. Maintaining integrity of the plan within changing circumstances of the environment is a critical aspect of any modification required.

The budget, particularly for those working as external evaluators, needs to be reviewed on a regular basis. If costs begin to exceed initial estimates, the evaluator needs to consider options for reducing expenses. Furthermore, these options should be discussed with key stakeholders.

Similarly, the schedule must be tracked to make certain that the project will be completed on time. In some organizations, the information from an evaluation will be used to make critical decisions. If the evaluation is not completed within schedule, decision makers will probably proceed to make the decision, and the evaluation findings may prove useless.

Effective evaluators identify and resolve problems quickly, whether the problems involve the budget, the schedule, or personnel. Some of these problems can involve conflicts among stakeholders, delays in data collection, inaccessibility of certain interviewees, and changes in key staff. A useful tool involves the development of a list of possible problems and possible solutions in the early stages of a project. Such a listing can aid the evaluator in making needed decisions to accomplish the tasks.

Fostering reflection and dialogue on the evaluation can be helpful to the evaluator, the evaluation team members, and the various stakeholders. It helps to identify the areas that proceeded successfully and the areas that provided challenges. This dialogue and reflection enable the various parties to learn from the evaluation so that future evaluation work can be improved.

14. Work effectively with personnel and stakeholders. This competency includes the following five performance standards:

    a) Manage team members, consultants, and technical experts.

    b) Keep stakeholders informed of progress.

    c) Keep the evaluation team engaged in and informed of the progress.

    d) Debrief evaluation team and stakeholders to establish lessons learned.

    e) Assess stakeholder satisfaction with the evaluation.

Evaluation is a participatory process, and management of such projects requires that evaluation specialists have personnel management, reporting, communication, and project assessment competencies. Of particular importance is developing skill sets in facilitative and collaborative approaches to management that engage all personnel and stakeholders in the right tasks, at the right time, according to the established plan. This includes all team members being informed of progress, sharing lessons learned, and openly and honestly providing assessment of their satisfaction with the evaluation process. Developing a management philosophy that is facilitative and collaborative is key to facilitating a successful evaluation process.

An effective evaluator early in a project establishes with stakeholders how much they want to be informed. In some cases, this will be weekly; in other cases, monthly or quarterly; and in still other cases, only at the end of the project. If someone wants to be kept informed on a regular basis, then the evaluator must create plans that allow for that level of reporting. At the same time, the evaluator must establish the kinds of stakeholder involvement needed for the project to progress successfully.

Some evaluations involve only the evaluator. In other situations, the evaluator becomes engaged in the issue of managing diverse groups of people and keeping them informed and on task. The larger the team, the more potential there is for communication breakdown and misunderstandings. This is a particular problem when the evaluation involves internal technical experts. In these cases, the evaluator must continually communicate that the project is a high priority when, to these experts (e.g., the IT specialists charged with uploading a survey), it is just "one more thing to do."

At the end of the evaluation, it is important for the evaluator to assess the evaluation effort itself (metaevaluation). Whether undertaken alone or as a team, there needs to be time for reflecting on the evaluation— what went well, what did not. Where were problems encountered that should have been anticipated and avoided? What should be done differently next time? Were stakeholders engaged as much as they needed to be? Ultimately, the evaluator has to answer the question, *Are the stakeholders fully satisfied with how this evaluation was conducted, the timeliness of it, and the quality of the report, irrespective of whether they like the findings and agree with the recommendations?*

CONCLUSIONS

The competencies needed by an evaluator cover a wide range of skills, knowledge, abilities, and attitudes. The first domain, *Professional Foundations,* involves competencies and features performance statements similar to other professional roles, such as training manager, instructional designer, and instructor. Similarly, the last domain, *Managing the Evaluation,* showcases skills, knowledge, abilities, and attitudes that are relevant for others who are involved in project management work. The domains of *Planning and Designing the Evaluation* and of *Implementing the Evaluation Plan* represent those competencies and performance statements that most evaluators would consider critical to the profession. Nevertheless, a competent evaluator must become familiar with all of these competencies and performance statements.

QUESTIONS FOR CONSIDERATION

Which of the competencies, in your view, are essential to all practitioner evaluators?

What competencies and performance standards are most applicable in your organization or in specific types of organizations?

What competencies and performance standards are least critical in your organization or in specific types of organizations? Why?

How would you go about applying the ibstpi Evaluator Competency model in your organization?

What resources or evidence would you suggest be included in a personal or organizational portfolio to demonstrate evaluation competencies at an individual or organizational level?

Are any of the competencies or performance statements likely to be affected by cross-cultural factors? If so, which ones?

CHAPTER

5

USE OF THE EVALUATOR COMPETENCIES

This chapter will enable you to accomplish the following:

- Describe how the ibstpi Evaluator Competency model can be used by those new to evaluation

- Describe how the Evaluator Competency model can be used by those who are experienced in evaluation

- Describe how the competency model can be used by those who manage training and development, human resources development and related functions, and evaluators in their work

- Describe how the Evaluator Competency model can be used by organizations such as academic institutions, consultants, and professional associations interested in providing development for evaluators

- Distinguish between certificate programs and certification

The evaluator competencies provide more than a description of the knowledge, skills, and abilities needed by someone undertaking an evaluation within an organizational setting. They present the job requirements for such individuals and, thus, can be used to develop position descriptions. Furthermore, these job requirements transcend place and cultural boundaries; given the increasing rate of globalization, it may be important for certain evaluators to be able to function across several different cultures. Competency listings in general, and these Evaluator Standards in particular, can give guidance to those who may be new to evaluation as well as those who are veterans in the field.

Both individuals and organizations can make use of these competencies. Practicing evaluators are the primary audience for these standards, which provide a benchmark against which to assess their knowledge and skill. For novices, such a benchmark will identify areas needing attention in order to develop greater evaluation expertise. For experienced practitioners, it will highlight areas for future specialization.

A secondary audience consists of managers who may be directing the work of an evaluator. Such persons will also find that these standards provide a useful set of guidelines when recruiting an evaluator either from within the organization or externally.

A third audience consists of the academic community. The standards provide a basis for developing evaluation courses within training and development (T&D) or human resource development (HRD) programs. These disciplines attract many students who expect to engage in evaluation activities in their future work. In addition to these specific disciplines, the ibstpi Evaluator Standards are relevant for any course of study where evaluation is a major task that graduates will undertake once they become professionals in the field.

Finally, professional associations and training consultants who provide professional development for T&D and HRD staff and other fields needing skills in evaluation can base their offerings around these competencies. Seminars on how to plan an evaluation, how to design and validate survey tools, or how to do content analysis of interview and focus group data are examples of professional development offerings based on the ibstpi standards. In addition, some professional organizations are considering the issue of certification for evaluators, and these standards can provide guidance here.

The following paragraphs will describe in greater depth the uses of the competencies by the four audiences. Each of the sections will end with a series of questions that should be asked by these individuals or groups.

COMPETENCY USE BY THOSE NEW TO EVALUATION

Many individuals within organizations, particularly within T&D or HRD, are required to undertake evaluation but do not possess academic training in the field. They have had to take on evaluation projects with little or no training, knowledge, or experience. That is why this book is important: it provides a detailed analysis of each competency as well as guidelines about how to use them to develop greater expertise. Thus, the ibstpi Evaluator Competency Standards are a useful tool in a variety of settings.

Many individuals whose primary role may be as a training manager, an instructional designer, an instructor, or an internal consultant are asked on occasion to undertake evaluation work, but they have no background or experience in evaluation. For such people, the standards provide essential concepts and terms as well as a window on the competencies required by their new evaluator role.

Depending on the job assignment, some competencies will be more relevant than others, but at a minimum, all evaluators, regardless of their level of experience, need to demonstrate competence in the professional foundations domain. Those with little or no experience with evaluations may find that they possess many of the competencies found in this domain. In the context of managing one's professional career, the Evaluator Competencies can also be used as a framework for organizing a personal log or professional portfolio representing the advancement of professional experience and interests. They may also choose to use the standards when hiring consultants, thereby ensuring that an external evaluator has the necessary skills to complement those of an internal evaluator. Similarly, training or HR practitioners who become interested in evaluation may use the standards to get an overview of the evaluation field and insight on the knowledge and skills required for effective evaluation.

Questions for Those New to Evaluation

- Which competencies or performance statements are required by my current job assignment?

- In which competencies am I weak or underdeveloped?

- How can I develop these competencies, or should some specific tasks be outsourced?

- Which competencies will be required for future work assignments or job opportunities?

COMPETENCY USE BY EXPERIENCED EVALUATORS

The standards can also be beneficial for those more experienced in evaluation. These are individuals who have undertaken several different evaluation efforts and usually possess some background education in the field. They conduct evaluations on a regular basis, possibly even as the major component of their job role.

Depending on their position and the amount of evaluation that they undertake, experienced evaluators may consider specializing or moving into a different evaluation role. A practitioner may move from designing postcourse evaluation surveys to developing expertise in focus groups and interviews. Similarly, an evaluator who has focused on formative evaluation to improve programs may want to learn how to measure the long-term effects of a program. The standards can help to identify the competencies needed to fill the specialized role and provide a blueprint for professional development.

The standards can also help evaluators or those undertaking evaluations in their quest to raise the quality of their practice and add to their competitive edge through professional development. By using the standards as a means of assessing personal skill gaps, it is possible to identify the appropriate courses targeting specific competencies. This also facilitates recognizing peers with complementary competencies and other potential resources for assistance. Conversely, by being aware of their assets, experienced evaluators can determine where they can contribute most to a project.

Among the performance statements that may draw the attention of evaluators looking to keep abreast of technological and methodological changes in their field are the following: *Stay current with new thinking and approaches in evaluation; Update one's professional skills; Stay current with relevant technology.* Reading the latest books and journals can help practitioners stay current with new ideas. Participation in online communities of practice as well as available conferences or workshops can aid individuals in their awareness of new approaches and new technologies.

For practitioners who undertake evaluation as part of their job role, the standards can be helpful when asking the question, *What are my areas of proficiency, and where do I need to further develop competence?* By assessing current areas of evaluation expertise, individuals can identify competencies that would improve their practice.

As in other professions, experienced evaluators are challenged by constant evolution and changes in the field. The ibstpi standards represent the state-of-the-art knowledge, skills, and attitudes of evaluators. Furthermore, the competencies and performance statements can be used as a guide to keeping up with evolving demands and talent needs at organizational and societal levels.

At the end of a project, the collection of competencies and performance statements can serve as a basis for metaevaluation or reflective practice. They can provide insight on an evaluator's own performance and identify skills that would have improved the evaluator's performance had they been stronger.

Questions for Experienced Evaluators

- Which competencies represent my proficiency as an evaluator?

- In which competencies am I weak or in need of improvement for the present project?

- Which competencies will be required for future work assignments or job opportunities?

- How can I develop the competencies that need improvement or that will be required in future work?

- Which competencies will be key to the success of this project?

- Which other competencies will enhance the success of this project?

COMPETENCY USE BY MANAGERS

Those managing T&D, HRD, and related functions within organizations can make use of the Evaluator Competencies. They can be used in managing individuals as well as teams and groups.

Managing Individuals

There exist numerous ways in which the Evaluator Competencies can be used in managing individuals. They can serve as the basis for developing or refining a job description for staff members who undertake evaluations. Similarly, these competencies or the resulting job descriptions can be used to recruit or hire new staff members, particularly when the position involves evaluation activities. Furthermore, they provide some guidelines for staff members, whether reassigned or newly hired, as to the expectations and competencies needed for the position.

In a similar manner, the competencies can also serve as the basis for selecting external evaluators. Because many managers may feel that the evaluation function is so specialized, they may choose to hire an external consultant to undertake evaluation efforts. Although several university programs exist to train evaluators, most of these focus on large-scale evaluation work. As a consequence, a savvy manager will need to explore the extent to which an external evaluator is familiar with the dynamics of undertaking an evaluation within an organizational setting; the ibstpi Evaluator Competencies can aid managers in making such a determination.

Whether dealing with internal staff or with an external consultant, managers can use the competencies to provide specific feedback to evaluators. For internal staff members, the competencies can aid managers in undertaking performance appraisals, mentoring, and coaching. Furthermore, they can help managers to identify training, education, and professional development needed by staff members to enhance their competencies. For external consultants, the competencies can aid managers in assessing the quality of the evaluation work being undertaken and in providing critical feedback, if needed.

Managing Teams and Groups

Although most evaluation efforts within organizational settings tend to be undertaken by an individual, there may be instances of larger-scale evaluations involving an evaluation team. The Evaluator Competencies can be used to identify the appropriate individuals needed for the project team. Team members can be selected to represent the range of competencies needed for the project. In addition, the competencies can be used to determine whether an external consultant should be employed to enhance the expertise of the team.

Having developed a project team, the manager can use the competencies as a guide when monitoring the work of the team and to provide team feedback. Such monitoring and feedback can help to identify when additional resources or additional mentoring, coaching, or development may be needed. At the conclusion of the project, the manager can adapt the competencies so as to provide a form of metaevaluation or reflection on the evaluation effort, which may elicit important lessons learned.

Questions for Those Managing or Recruiting Evaluators

- Do the job descriptions of those individuals or teams being tasked with an evaluation reflect the range of competencies required?

- Do current employees demonstrate the competencies needed to undertake an evaluation?

- Does the prospective employee have the competencies needed to undertake an evaluation?

- Do the competencies of the prospective employee complement those of the department or team?

- Has the prospective consultant provided evidence of competence in the specific needed areas?

- What interventions are needed to improve the competencies of those involved in the evaluation work?

COMPETENCY USE IN ACADEMIC SETTINGS

The ibstpi Evaluator Competencies can be a useful tool for those who prepare future evaluators. Many colleges and universities offer courses that focus on evaluation. Outstanding evaluation programs are organizationally focused and grounded in the theory and practice of evaluation. The ibstpi Evaluator Competencies provide a reliable basis for determining these needs because of their currency, comprehensive scope of evaluator responsibilities, applicability to a broad range of organizations where evaluation work is conducted, and practitioner-based data that attest to their validation on a global scale. Thus, these standards can serve as a guide for academic curriculum development and program revisions, accreditation processes, and forming research agendas.

Developing and Updating Evaluation Curricula

The most comprehensive preparation of evaluation specialists generally takes place in graduate university programs. These programs are shaped to a great extent by the skills needed in the marketplace, literature about the evaluation field, ideas from professional organizations, and the capabilities, experiences, and vision of the faculty. The standards provide a useful tool for identifying the skills and knowledge needed in the workplace.

The Evaluation Competency domains (e.g., *Professional Foundations, Planning and Designing the Evaluation*, etc.) and the competencies themselves can serve as a framework to construct and update an evaluation program. Competency domains may also lend themselves to the process of constructing courses. The *Professional Foundations* domain, for example, may be especially pertinent to introductory courses. The *Planning and Designing Evaluation* and *Implementing Evaluation* domains are relevant to in-depth evaluation process courses. The *Managing Evaluation* domain may be pertinent to both basic and advanced courses. In basic courses, certain of the critical management skills relevant to positions throughout an organization could be introduced. More advanced courses could emphasize specific skills needed for those focused on the management of evaluation projects.

The competencies and performance statements can also be used as a basis to review and revise existing curricula, typically an ongoing task in academia. The competencies can be used to assess a program's currency, completeness, depth of course content, and integration of appropriate practice activities. This review can, then, be incorporated into the program's self-study materials when needed.

The performance statements can serve as course objectives that inform course content and practice activities, particularly as related to evaluation courses and programs. They can also form the basis for portfolios and other forms of assessment of students in evaluation programs. Preskill and Russ-Eft (2005), for example, include a number of similar activities for building evaluation capacity.

Finally, the ibstpi competencies can be used by faculty to guide and mentor students who are interested in careers in training or human resources that use evaluation. Both faculty and students can decide whether courses, internships, and other experiences will aid in developing the needed competencies for such careers. The box titled "Questions for University Faculty Reviewing Evaluation Program Curricula" presents questions for those teaching, developing, or revising academic programs in evaluation.

Accrediting Evaluation Programs

Most academic programs must conduct periodic self-studies and be reviewed by internal and external accrediting bodies. Although such bodies typically have general guidelines and standards to which the department must respond, it is often left to the program to identify more specific criteria that directly address their mission. Chosen standards,

Questions for University Faculty Reviewing Evaluation Program Curricula

- To what extent does the curriculum address each of the competency domain areas?

- To what extent does the curriculum content address each of the competencies and performance standards?

- Are there adequate practice activities to address all of the competencies and performance standards?

- Are students introduced to the ibstpi Evaluator Competencies as a way to track their own development?

- How effectively are the competencies used to advise students who are interested in preparing for training, HR, or human performance careers that use evaluation?

- How effectively are the competencies used to guide the placement of students in relevant internships and work-study programs?

- To what extent does the curriculum address the professional development needs of graduate students currently working as training or evaluation specialists?

- How many additional faculty are needed to increase the number of courses required to adequately address the range of competencies needed in the current market?

however, must be authoritative and valid for each field. Departments that offer evaluation curricula can use the ibstpi Evaluation Competencies to analyze and document their programs and to assess curriculum content and progress in student proficiency. In this way, the competencies can be a basis for benchmarking best evaluation practices.

Assessing Student Performance

In addition to their use in examining academic programs and courses, the ibstpi competencies can also be used to assess student performance. Because these are the competencies considered essential by those engaged in this work, students should be expected to become familiar with the competencies and to demonstrate their own level of competence. Various approaches exist to assess student performance, including tests, demonstrations, practicums, and internships. Portfolios represent another approach, and the competencies can serve as the basis for the development of student portfolios demonstrating students' knowledge and competence with all or some of the Evaluator Competencies.

Forming Research Agendas

Much academic work focuses on research. Whereas research agendas are largely dependent on individual interests and expertise, the ibstpi Evaluator Competencies can provide some direction to research plans. These competencies identify the scope and emphasis of current evaluation practices. They provide a comprehensive list of topics and skills important to practicing professionals. Research addressing any of the topics is more likely to be attuned to the concerns and needs of the practitioner communities.

Specific research areas and questions suggested by the ibstpi standards include the following:

- How do societal, business, and technological changes impact the evolution of these Evaluator or Competencies?

- What is the relationship, if any, between organizational size and culture on the competency profiles of evaluators?

- To what extent are emerging technologies changing the practice of evaluation and reprioritizing the competencies?

The ibstpi Evaluator Competencies have a high degree of credibility in the T&D, HRD, and performance improvement professions. Aligning curriculum or individual evaluation courses with these standards ensures that students are receiving a balanced and wide-ranging coverage of the tasks of a professional evaluator. Academic programs that align their curriculum with the standards can be confident that they are providing instruction most likely to develop the capabilities required of evaluators in the work environment.

USE BY CONSULTANTS PROVIDING EVALUATION SEMINARS

Not all of those undertaking evaluations within organizational settings have received formal education in evaluation courses or programs. This was confirmed by the research conducted to validate these competencies.

The expertise of many of these "evaluators" has been developed on the job while they were employed as a trainer, instructional designer, HR professional, or a training manager. In other cases, individuals have received formal education courses or degrees in program evaluation, typically with a focus on large-scale government-funded evaluation, but they have found themselves working within an organizational setting. Both of these groups have typically supplemented their knowledge and skills by attending professional workshops and seminars.

Training consultants, both individual providers and members of large consulting firms, offer general as well as customized workshops in evaluation. Such consultants should find the competency standards to be valuable as a basis for developing and enhancing their offerings. They can use the competencies and performance statements in much the same way as academic faculty as a means to ensure that their content encompasses the key skills and areas of knowledge. Such courses can be broad in their coverage of the competencies, or they can focus on specific areas, such as how to develop an effective evaluation plan or how to analyze and interpret data. The broad acceptance of the ibstpi standards within the HRD and T&D fields adds to the credibility of workshops and seminars based on the competencies. Questions in the box titled "Questions for Training Consultants" may be helpful to evaluation consultants in developing relevant professional development seminars and programs.

Questions for Training Consultants

- Are the development opportunities tailored to the needs of practitioners without formal qualifications as evaluators?

- Are offerings clearly identifiable as novice or experienced?

- Do the offerings focus on the competencies in which practitioners typically do not perform well?

- Do workshops or seminars provide opportunity for practice and feedback?

- Are the seminars available online for those who wish to do distance education?

- How are attendees assessed to confirm proficiency in the competencies?

COMPETENCY USE BY ASSOCIATIONS

The ibstpi competencies are also attractive to large and small professional associations with which today's training, HRD, and performance improvement professionals are affiliated. One important area of concern for such associations is that of providing professional development opportunities. Thus, they can use the ibstpi Evaluator Competencies, as described in the previous section on use by consultants providing evaluation seminars, to help determine the content areas that may be needed by association members.

A second area of interest for some associations is *certification.* Certification is a designation that assures that someone is qualified to perform a job. According to the certifying body, the individual has demonstrated knowledge, skills, or abilities to a specified standard. As important, certification may be distinguished from being *credentialed, degreed, accredited,* or *licensed* (or all of these)—although the lines between and among these designations are increasingly blurred.

Although associations vary dramatically in structure, reach, number or type of members, membership qualifications, fees, and services or products, common to them is a move to support or internally develop sets of competencies that attend to the major functional areas in which their members work. In some cases, these competencies are linked to learning programs where certificates are awarded to attendees who finish one or more courses of study but are not tested. Such programs differ from certification, in which attendees complete prescribed courses of study *and* pass one or more qualifying examinations. Formal certification programs are organized around domains or performance or behavioral standards about which experts agree and are marketed as a way to attest that successful completers are better qualified for specific tasks and responsibilities than those trained solely on the job or through more informal means (Hale, 2000). Associations seeking to integrate the ibstpi Evaluator Competencies into a certification process will find a well-crafted, thoughtfully developed set of skills, knowledge, and aptitudes with which to work.

The ibstpi Evaluator Competencies can also be applied less formally in certificate programs or other growth options that organizations or professional groups provide to members. Why? Because these competencies attend well to the several evaluation domains (planning, implementing, managing, and analyzing or reporting) that are critical to evaluation work and yet peripheral or ancillary to the work these people do; evaluation simply is not the primary focus of their job.

Given the growing importance of professional associations among workplace professionals, some examples will be provided of ways such groups can grow or broaden competency-based programs. The American Society for Training and Development (ASTD) and the International Society for Performance Improvement (ISPI) currently have certificate and certification programs. These associations could use the ibstpi Evaluator Competencies to enhance the professional development and certification focused on evaluation activities. Similarly, other professional associations that focus on trainers and instructors, instructional designers, and organizational development continue to examine evaluation issues, and these associations could use the competencies to enhance their offerings. Finally, the myriad national and regional evaluation-related associations could incorporate the ibstpi competencies to enhance the development opportunities for members who focus on organizational evaluations.

In summary, then, professional associations that embrace the ibstpi Evaluator Competencies, whether as part of certification or through more informal learning opportunities, should consider both the *association* and *personal* benefits of their adoption or adaptation.

The following are some association benefits:

- To ensure that the association is prepared for an ever-changing marketplace

- To illustrate the association's commitment to quality and high performance and its members' specialized expertise

- To illustrate the association's focus on member satisfaction—specifically, its ability to meet member needs

- To suggest that the association has firmly established performance expectations

- To suggest that the association attends to professional growth and development

- To decrease turnover or attrition of members

  Personal benefits (to members) would include the following:

- To suggest a level of competence that sets the individual apart from others

- To set performance expectations

- To strengthen career advancement opportunities

- To build confidence

CONCLUSIONS

The ibstpi Evaluator Competencies can be used at both the individual and organizational or institutional levels. Individuals, for example, might turn to them to improve personal competence, identify appropriate individuals for undertaking a project, or select individual consultants who will design and facilitate training and workshops on evaluation-related issues. Universities, on the other hand, might use them to develop and improve their research, assessment, or evaluation courses, whereas professional associations may build evaluation training or certification programs around them. In all cases, the ibstpi Evaluator Competencies identify what is needed currently by evaluators as well as what will be needed in the future.

QUESTIONS FOR CONSIDERATION

Which types of use of the ibstpi Evaluator Competency model are of most interest to you personally?

Which types of use are of most interest to your organization or institution?

What other types of use might need to be considered?

Which areas of development need are highlighted for you (using the lists of questions), and how will you develop those competency areas?

PART

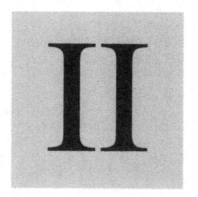

II

THE IBSTPI EVALUATOR COMPETENCIES: VALIDATION

CHAPTER 6

SOME FOUNDATIONAL RESEARCH

This chapter will enable you to accomplish the following:

- Describe the various ethical standards and guidelines informing the ibstpi Evaluator Competencies work

- Describe previously completed studies that form a foundation for the ibstpi Evaluator Competencies

- Recognize the importance of the various standards and ethical guidelines that exist throughout the world

The ibstpi Evaluator Competencies are empirically based and empirically validated. They are grounded in previous research efforts and are based on the ibstpi process for developing and validating these competencies, as outlined in Chapter 3. In this chapter, we review the specific studies and work representing the foundational research.

THE FOUNDATIONAL RESEARCH

The work that formed the foundation for the development of the ibstpi Evaluator Competencies included the following:

- The *Program Evaluation Standards* by the Joint Committee on Standards for Educational Evaluation (1994)

- The *Guiding Principles for Evaluators* by the American Evaluation Association (1995, revised in 2004)

- The *CES Guidelines for Ethical Conduct* by the Canadian Evaluation Society (2003)

- The *Standards für Evaluation* by the Deutsche Gesellschaft für Evaluation (2001)

- The *Guidelines for the Ethical Conduct of Evaluations* (2006) and the "Code of Ethics" (no date) of the Australasian Evaluation Society

- The *Standards on Ethics and Integrity* by the Academy of Human Resource Development (1999)

- The King, Stevahn, Ghere, and Minnema work (King et al., 2001; Ghere et al., 2006; Stevahn et al., 2005, 2006) on essential program evaluator competencies

- The Engle, Altschuld, and Kim (2006) survey of university-based evaluation programs. We also sought competency lists from academic programs in universities in the United States, Canada, Europe, and Australia.

Each of these will be described briefly.

THE PROGRAM EVALUATION STANDARDS

The following section describes the purpose and procedures used to develop the Program Evaluation Standards. We then discuss the results and the application of those standards in the work by the ibstpi team.

Purpose and Procedures

During the 1974 revision of the *Standards for Educational and Psychological Tests and Manuals,* issues arose concerning the use of tests in the evaluation of educational programs. The committee working on those standards, which included members of the American Educational Research Association, the American Psychological Association, and the National Council on Measurement in Education, decided that resolving these issues required a new committee. In 1975, the committee from these three organizations recommended that their committee be expanded in membership and that this larger committee develop standards for educational evaluation. The committee, named the Joint Committee, eventually included members from 12 organizations. The Joint Committee used a public process for the development of its standards. This process included experts in evaluation, users of evaluation, and those interested in the quality of educational evaluation. This public process included a panel of writers, review panels, field test sites, public hearings, a validation panel, and review by the Joint Committee and interested critics. Their work resulted in the publication of *Standards for Evaluations of Educational Programs, Projects, and Materials* (1981). Two specific areas were not included: evaluation of institutions because of accreditation agency work, and personnel evaluation, which was later undertaken as a separate effort by the Joint Committee.

The Joint Committee was incorporated as a nonprofit entity in 1981, with the purpose of developing and promoting evaluation standards. Then in 1989, the American National Standards Institute (ANSI) accredited the Joint Committee's process for developing standards. During that same year, the Joint Committee decided to reexamine its 1981 standards because of an increasing interest by those working beyond school settings to use these standards. The *Program Evaluation Standards* (Joint Committee on Standards for Educational Evaluation, 1994) resulted from a thorough review process and includes illustrations and applications from "schools, universities, law, medicine, nursing, the military, business, government, and social service agencies" (p. xvii).

Results

The standards are organized around four areas: utility, feasibility, propriety, and accuracy as described in the following box.

The Program Evaluation Standards

Utility

The utility standards are intended to ensure that an evaluation will serve the information needs of intended users.

U1 **Stakeholder identification.** Persons involved in or affected by the evaluation should be identified so that their needs can be addressed.

(Continued)

U2 **Evaluator credibility.** The persons conducting the evaluation should be both trustworthy and competent to perform the evaluation so that the evaluation findings achieve maximum credibility and acceptance.

U3 **Information scope and selection.** Information collected should be broadly selected to address pertinent questions about the program and be responsive to the needs and interests of clients and other specified stakeholders.

U4 **Values identification.** The perspectives, procedures, and rationale used to interpret the findings should be carefully described so that the bases for value judgments are clear.

U5 **Report clarity.** Evaluation reports should clearly describe the program being evaluated, including its context and the purposes, procedures, and findings of the evaluation so that essential information is provided and easily understood.

U6 **Report timeliness and dissemination.** Significant interim findings and evaluation reports should be disseminated to intended users so that they can be used in a timely fashion.

U7 **Evaluation impact.** Evaluations should be planned, conducted, and reported in ways that encourage follow-through by stakeholders so that the likelihood that the evaluation will be used is increased.

Feasibility

The feasibility standards are intended to ensure that an evaluation will be practical, realistic, prudent, diplomatic, and frugal.

F1 **Practical procedures.** The evaluation procedures should be practical to keep disruption to a minimum while needed information is obtained.

F2 **Political viability.** The evaluation should be planned and conducted with anticipation of the different positions of various interest groups so that their cooperation may be obtained and so that possible attempts by any of these groups to curtail evaluation operations or to bias or misapply the results can be averted or counteracted.

F3 **Cost-effectiveness.** The evaluation should be efficient and produce information of sufficient value that the resources expended can be justified.

Propriety

The propriety standards are intended to ensure that an evaluation will be conducted legally, ethically, and with due regard for the welfare of those involved in the evaluation as well as those affected by its results.

PI **Service orientation.** Evaluations should be designed to assist organizations to address and effectively serve the needs of the full range of targeted participants.

P2 **Formal agreements.** Obligations of the formal parties to an evaluation (what is to be done, how, by whom, when) should be agreed to in writing so that these parties are obligated to adhere to all conditions of the agreement or formally to renegotiate it.

P3 **Rights of human subjects.** Evaluations should be designed and conducted to respect and protect the rights and welfare of human subjects.

P4 **Human interactions.** Evaluators should respect human dignity and worth in their interactions with other persons associated with an evaluation so that participants are not threatened or harmed.

P5 **Complete and fair assessment.** The evaluation should be complete and fair in its examination and recording of strengths and weaknesses of the program being evaluated so that strengths can be built upon and problem areas addressed.

P6 **Disclosure of findings.** The formal parties to an evaluation should ensure that the full set of evaluation findings, along with pertinent limitations, are made accessible to the persons affected by the evaluation and any others with expressed legal rights to receive the results.

P7 **Conflict of interest.** Conflict of interest should be dealt with openly and honestly, so that it does not compromise the evaluation processes and results.

P8 **Fiscal responsibility.** The evaluator's allocation and expenditure of resources should reflect sound accountability procedures and otherwise be prudent and ethically responsible so that expenditures are accounted for and appropriate.

(Continued)

Accuracy

The accuracy standards are intended to ensure that an evaluation will reveal and convey technically adequate information about the features that determine worth of merit of the program being evaluated.

Al **Program documentation.** The program being evaluated should be described and documented clearly and accurately so that the program is clearly identified.

A2 **Context analysis.** The context in which the program exists should be examined in enough detail that its likely influences on the program can be identified.

A3 **Described purposes and procedures.** The purposes and procedures of the evaluation should be monitored and described in enough detail that they can be identified and assessed.

A4 **Defensible information sources.** The sources of information used in a program evaluation should be described in enough detail that the adequacy of the information can be assessed.

A5 **Valid information.** The information-gathering procedures should be chosen or developed and then implemented so that they will assure that the interpretation arrived at is valid for the intended use.

A6 **Reliable information.** The information-gathering procedures should be chosen or developed and then implemented so that they will assure that the information obtained is sufficiently reliable for the intended use.

A7 **Systematic information.** The information collected, processed, and reported in an evaluation should be systematically reviewed, and any errors found should be corrected.

A8 **Analysis of quantitative information.** Quantitative information in an evaluation should be appropriately and systematically analyzed so that evaluation questions are effectively answered.

A9 **Analysis of qualitative information.** Qualitative information in an evaluation should be appropriately and systematically analyzed so that evaluation questions are effectively answered.

A10 **Justified conclusions.** The conclusions reached in an evaluation should be explicitly justified so that stakeholders can assess them.

A11 **Impartial reporting.** Reporting procedures should guard against distortion caused by personal feelings and biases of any party to the evaluation so that evaluation reports fairly reflect the evaluation findings.

A12 **Metaevaluation.** The evaluation itself should be formatively and summatively evaluated against these and other pertinent standards so that its conduct is appropriately guided and, on completion, stakeholders can closely examine its strengths and weaknesses.

Reproduced with permission from the Joint Committee on Standards for Educational Evaluation.

Application of These Standards

Given the wide use of these standards worldwide, the ibstpi Evaluator Competencies group carefully reviewed the standards for their applicability to our target audience—that is, evaluators working within organizational settings. The use of these standards is reflected in several of the competencies, such as 2, *Establish and maintain professional credibility,* and 4, *Observe ethical and legal standards* (see Chapters 3 and 4).

GUIDING PRINCIPLES BY THE AMERICAN EVALUATION ASSOCIATION

In the following section, we describe the purpose for the development of the guiding principles and procedures used in their development. We then discuss the results and the application of those standards in the work by the ibstpi team.

Purpose and Procedures

The American Evaluation Association (AEA) was formed in 1985 as a union of two separate evaluation organizations: the Evaluation Network and the Evaluation Research Society. Recognizing the need for a professional association to develop a set of ethical guidelines, an AEA task force was commissioned to create a set of guidelines or standards. The task force agreed that its work should complement rather than compete with the *Program Evaluation Standards.* Their work resulted in the *Guiding Principles for Evaluators* (American Evaluation Association, 1995). More recently, a similar AEA task force revisited the *Guiding Principles for Evaluators,* and those principles were ratified during the business meeting of the association (American Evaluation Association, 2004).

Results

The *Guiding Principles for Evaluators* identifies five principles (reproduced here with AEA's permission):

- *Systematic inquiry:* Evaluators conduct systematic, data-based inquiries.

- *Competence:* Evaluators provide competent performance to stakeholders.

- *Integrity and honesty:* Evaluators display honesty and integrity in their own behavior and attempt to ensure the honesty and integrity of the entire evaluation process.

- *Respect for people:* Evaluators respect the security, dignity, and self-worth of the respondents, program participants, clients, and other stakeholders.

- *Responsibilities for the general and public welfare:* Evaluators articulate and take into account the diversity of general and public interests and values that may be related to the evaluation.

Application of These Principles

The ibstpi team reviewed the principles to identify where it was appropriate to integrate them into the ibstpi competencies in some form. Certainly the work of the ibstpi team is directed toward enhancing the competence of those who perform evaluations within organizations. In addition, systematic inquiry, integrity and honesty, and respect for people are included within the Evaluator Competencies. The last guiding principle—responsibilities for the general and public welfare—appeared to be relevant to certain types of evaluations and certain kinds of organizations, but it did not suggest a particular competency needed by those working within organizational settings.

GUIDELINES FOR ETHICAL CONDUCT BY THE CANADIAN EVALUATION SOCIETY

We next describe the purpose for the development of the Canadian Evaluation Society (CES) *Guidelines for Ethical Conduct* and procedures used in their development. We then discuss the results and the creation of professional development seminars called Essential Skills, as well as a core body of knowledge (CBK) for program evaluation. The section ends with a description of the application of those standards in the work by the ibstpi team.

Purpose and Procedures

Beginning in 1988 and 1989, the CES, both with a national committee and its chapters, explored the issue of ethical guidelines. These groups advocated for nonprescriptive guidelines. A discussion paper by Marthe Hurteau, "Reflections on a Code of Ethics" (1993), revisited the issue, and the paper was discussed by the various chapters. A working group refined the guidelines and presented a session at the annual CES National Conference in Quebec in 1994. Based on the panel discussion and later assistance from the National Council Professional Development Committee, a questionnaire was circulated to the membership to obtain feedback and input. The final set of *Guidelines for Ethical Conduct* was published in 1996. Thus, CES decided to "promote its own set of ethical guidelines rather than to endorse guidelines produced by the American Evaluation Association (AEA)" (Keith, 2003, p. 13).

Results

The *CES Guidelines for Ethical Conduct* discuss competence, integrity, and accountability.

CES Guidelines for Ethical Conduct

Competence

Evaluators are to be competent in their provision of service.

1. Evaluators should apply systematic methods of inquiry appropriate to the evaluation.
2. Evaluators should possess or provide content knowledge appropriate for the evaluation.
3. Evaluators should continuously strive to improve their methodological and practice skills.

(Continued)

Integrity

Evaluators are to act with integrity in their relationships with all stakeholders.

1. Evaluators should accurately represent their level of skills and knowledge.

2. Evaluators should declare any conflict of interest to clients before embarking on an evaluation project and at any point where such conflict occurs. This includes conflict of interest on the part of either evaluator or stakeholder.

3. Evaluators should be sensitive to the cultural and social environment of all stakeholders and conduct themselves in a manner appropriate to this environment.

4. Evaluators should confer with the client on contractual decisions such as confidentiality, privacy, communication, and ownership of findings and reports.

Accountability

Evaluators are to be accountable for their performance and their product.

1. Evaluators should be responsible for the provision of information to clients to facilitate their decision-making concerning the selection of appropriate evaluation strategies and methodologies. Such information should include the limitations of selected methodology.

2. Evaluators should be responsible for the clear, accurate, and fair written and/or oral presentation of study findings and limitations, and recommendations.

3. Evaluators should be responsible in their fiscal decision-making so that expenditures are accounted for and clients receive good value for their dollars.

4. Evaluators should be responsible for the completion of the evaluation within a reasonable time as agreed to with the clients. Such agreements should acknowledge unprecedented delays resulting from factors beyond the evaluator's control.

These guidelines continue to be addressed in a series of professional development seminars called Essential Skills, which cover (1) understanding program evaluation, (2) building an evaluation framework, (3) improving program performance, and (4) evaluating for results. Furthermore, the CES has been engaged in the development of a Core Body of Knowledge (CBK) for program evaluation, and this work has identified the benefits, outputs, and knowledge elements listed in the box following (Zorzi, McGuire, & Perrin, 2002).

Potential Benefits

- Accountability
- Decision making
- Knowledge and skills
- Social change
- Cohesion and collaboration

Outputs

- Needs assessment outputs
- Evaluability assessment outputs
- Process evaluation outputs
- Outcome or impact evaluation outputs
- Efficiency assessment outputs
- Outputs of stakeholder involvement
- Outputs spanning all types of evaluation

Knowledge Elements

- Ethics
- Evaluation planning and design
- Data collection
- Data analysis and interpretation
- Communication and interpersonal skills
- Project management

Reproduced with permission of Zorzi, McGuirre, and Perrin.

Application of These Guidelines

The ibstpi group recognized that the guidelines supported our work in terms of the focus on competence and competencies. Furthermore, these guidelines helped to inform several of the performance statements, such as *2.c. Stay current with new thinking and approaches in evaluation and related fields.* Of greater importance and providing corroboration of the ibstpi competencies were the knowledge elements. Specifically, these appeared to align with the domains, such as *Planning and Designing the Evaluation* and *Managing the Evaluation.*

STANDARDS FÜR EVALUATION OF THE DEUTSCHE GESELLSCHAFT FÜR EVALUATION

In the following section, we describe the purpose for the standards, and the procedures used in their development. We then discuss the results and the application of those standards in the work by the ibstpi team.

Purpose and Procedures

The *Standards für Evaluation* of the Deutsche Gesellschaft für Evaluation (DeGEval) were inspired by the work of the Joint Committee, as described above, as well as the Swiss adaptation, "which provides a generalization of these standards from educational to more diverse settings" (Beywl & Taut, 2001, p. 1). The development involved the work of a standards committee of the DeGEval, a survey of the membership, and a review. This development process took two years; the Standards were ratified by the Society on October 4, 2001.

Results

Similar to the work of the Joint Committee, the standards were organized into four basic attributes: utility, feasibility, propriety, and accuracy.

Application of the Standards

The ibstpi group reviewed these standards but felt that the issues and concerns had been identified in the standards developed previously by the Joint Committee.

GUIDELINES FOR ETHICAL CONDUCT OF EVALUATIONS AND CODE OF ETHICS OF THE AUSTRALASIAN EVALUATION SOCIETY

In this section we describe the purpose for the development of the *Code of Ethics* and the *Guidelines for Ethical Conduct,* as well as procedures used in their development. We then discuss the results and the application of those standards in the work by the ibstpi team.

Purpose and Process

The Australasian Evaluation Society (AES) has developed both a *Code of Ethics* and *Guidelines for Ethical Conduct.* The purpose of the *Code of Ethics* is to provide "a statement of the values and principles which members uphold in their work in evaluation and in their membership of the Society" (Australasian Evaluation Society, n.d., paragraph 1). The code was adopted by the Society in December 2000.

After several years of development, AES's board endorsed the *Guidelines for Ethical Conduct* in 1997 and distributed them to the members in 1998. They were incorporated into the *Code of Ethics* in December 2000.

Results

The code includes both responsibilities to the field of evaluation and the public and responsibilities to the Society and the fellow members. Only the responsibilities to the field of evaluation and the public were considered relevant to ibstpi's work, and these are listed in the following box.

Responsibilities to the Field of Evaluation and to the Public

■ **Ethical conduct**: When commissioning, conducting, or reporting an evaluation, members should strive to uphold the ethical principles and associated procedures endorsed by the society in the *Guidelines for the Ethical Conduct of Evaluations*.

COMMISSIONING AND PREPARING FOR AN EVALUATION

- ■ Briefing document
- ■ Identify limitations and different interests
- ■ Contractual arrangement
- ■ Advise changing circumstances
- ■ Look for potential risks or harms
- ■ Practice within competence
- ■ Discuss potential conflict of interest
- ■ Compete honorably
- ■ Deal openly and fairly

CONDUCTING AN EVALUATION

- ■ Consider implications of differences and inequalities
- ■ Identify purpose and commissioners
- ■ Obtain informed consent
- ■ Be sufficiently rigorous
- ■ Declare limitations
- ■ Maintain confidentiality
- ■ Report significant problems
- ■ Anticipate serious wrongdoing

REPORTING THE RESULTS OF AN EVALUATION

- Report clearly and simply
- Report fairly and comprehensively
- Identify sources and make acknowledgments
- Fully reflect evaluator's findings
- Do not breach integrity of the reports

- **Public interest**
- **Quality work**
- **Compensation**
- **Courtesy**
- **Integrity**
- **Truthfulness**
- **Reasonable criticism**
- **Confidentiality**
- **Acknowledgment**
- **Introduction of work**

Reproduced with permission of the Australasian Evaluation Society.

Application of This Work

The *Guidelines for Ethical Conduct* proved most useful to ibstpi's work because it aided in the development of some of the major domains. So, for example, *Commissioning and Preparing the Evaluation* shows similarities to the domain of *Planning and Designing the Evaluation.*

STANDARDS ON ETHICS AND INTEGRITY BY THE ACADEMY OF HUMAN RESOURCE DEVELOPMENT

In the following section, we describe the purpose for the development of the standards and procedures used in their development. We then discuss the results and the application of those standards in the work by the ibstpi team.

Purpose and Procedures

The Academy of Human Resource Development (AHRD) began in 1994 and was formed to lead the profession through research. After several years as an association, members began to recognize the need for a set of ethical standards. A task force was formed to develop such a set. The process involved reviewing various sets of existing standards, including the *Program Evaluation Standards* and the AEA *Guiding Principles* as well as those of the Academy of Management, the American Educational Research Association, the American Psychological Association, and the Organizational Development Network. Adapting and expanding upon the various sets of standards, the task force developed an initial draft set, which was shared with the AHRD Board during one of its meetings and with the membership during an interactive session at one of the conferences. The final set of standards was adopted by the AHRD Board.

Results

The AHRD *Standards* recognize the varieties of ethical issues confronting human resource development researchers and practitioners. These standards included details on the following areas:

- General principles
- General standards
- Research and evaluation
- Advertising and other public statements
- Publication of work
- Privacy and confidentiality
- Resolution of ethical issues and violations

Application of the Standards

The ibstpi evaluation team reviewed the AHRD standards and recognized that only certain standards appeared applicable to the development of competencies for evaluators. Both the general principles and the specific section on research and evaluation provided relevance for the ibstpi work (see the following box).

General Principles

- Competence
- Integrity
- Professional responsibility
- Respect for people's rights and dignity
- Concern for others' welfare
- Social responsibility

General Standards

- Data collection
- Responsibility
- Compliance with the law and standards
- Institutional approval
- Informed consent
- Incentives to participants
- Deception in research
- Interpretation and explanation of research and evaluation results

Reproduced with permission of the Academy of Human Resource Development.

THE KING, STEVAHN, GHERE, AND MINNEMA WORK ON ESSENTIAL EVALUATOR COMPETENCIES

In the following section, we describe the purpose of this particular study and the procedures. We then discuss the results and the application of these results in the work by the ibstpi team.

Purpose and Procedures

This work began as an exploratory study to "determine the extent to which evaluation professionals, representing diverse backgrounds and approaches, could reach consensus on . . . essential evaluator competencies" (King, Stevahn, Ghere, & Minnema, 2001, p. 229). Graduate students involved in an evaluation course used a concept formation process to identify essential evaluator competencies. These were refined by the instructor and three of the graduate students using some of the standards mentioned above to prepare a draft listing of competencies. Two separate pilots of these competencies were undertaken with six evaluation professionals and two graduate students.

To measure the face validity, a procedure called Multi-Attribute Consensus Building was employed in which small groups of three to ten people (with a total participation of 31 people from the Minneapolis–St. Paul area) rated the importance of the competencies. The results were tabulated to show the extent of agreement or disagreement, followed by a period of discussion of the ratings. Then people provided their final ratings.

Additional work has continued to examine these essential competencies (Stevahn, King, Ghere, & Minnema, 2005) to determine their congruence with university evaluation programs (Stevahn et al., 2006) and to present a professional development unit for individuals to reflect on these competencies (Ghere, King, Stevahn, & Minnema, 2006).

Results

The original study identified the major competency areas, shown in the following box.

Major Competencies

I. Systematic Inquiry

   IA. Able to do research-oriented activities

   IB. Able to do evaluation-oriented activities

   IC. Able to do activities common to both research and evaluation

II. Competent Evaluation Practice

   IIA. Able to serve the information needs of intended users

   IIB. Able to do situational analysis

   IIC. Able to organize and manage evaluation projects

III. General Skills for Evaluation Practice

   IIIA. Logical and critical thinking skills

   IIIB. Written communication skills

   IIIC. Verbal communication skills

   IIID. Interpersonal competence

   IIIE. Computer application skills

IV. Evaluation Professionalism

   IVA. Knowledge of yourself as an evaluator

   IVB. Ethical conduct

   IVC. Knowledge of professional standards (e.g., Joint Committee Standards and AEA *Guiding Principles*)

   IVD. Application of professional standards

   IVE. Professional development

Application of This Research

The work of King and colleagues provided an important base for the initial development of the ibstpi competencies. They helped to identify a variety of different issues and competency areas common to all evaluation practice. At the same time, the team recognized that our work needed to go deeper into the specific competencies needed by those functioning within an organizational setting.

THE ENGLE, ALTSCHULD, AND KIM SURVEY OF UNIVERSITY-BASED EVALUATION PROGRAMS

We describe the purpose of this study and procedures used in the work by Engle, Altschuld, and Kim (2006). We then discuss the results and the application of these results by the ibstpi team.

Purpose and Procedures

The purpose of the study was to determine the nature of university programs that prepare people to become evaluators. Also, this particular study represented an update of a similar 1992 survey of such programs (Altschuld et al., 1994). The authors developed a listing of prospective respondent programs through a call-in EvalTalk (the AEA-sponsored electronic discussion), announcements at the 2000 AEA conference, requests for nominations from the AEA Board, and a review by the president of the CES. In addition, the researchers compared the listing with the 1992 listing. The sampling frame included 63 U.S.-based programs and 23 programs based in other countries. An e-mail requesting response through an online survey was sent to individuals identified as the primary contact person for each of the programs. Thirty-eight completed surveys were received, with 27 from the United States, six from Canada, one from Australia, and one each from Iceland, Belgium, and the West Indies.

Results

A rank ordering of program goals showed that the highest-ranked goal across all of the programs involved conducting evaluations of programs or projects. The most frequently mentioned courses included in these programs were

- Evaluation project or research

- Introduction to evaluation

- Models or theories of evaluation

- Program evaluation

- Applied evaluation

Application of This Research

Although the specific results of this survey were not available at the beginning of the ibstpi Evaluator Competencies work, the team did gather available syllabi from evaluation courses and programs. This data gathering was not as thorough and systematic as the Engle, Altschuld, and Kim survey, but it yielded similar results, specifically in terms of the most common courses. Furthermore, the ibstpi Evaluator Competencies team undertook a thorough review of the course syllabi to identify relevant competencies for inclusion in the initial drafting.

CONCLUSIONS

Evaluation as a profession has recently matured, and with it, various national evaluation association and related entities have undertaken the development of standards and guidelines for evaluators. In addition, evaluation experts themselves have recognized the need for the development of professional competencies. The work described in this chapter helps to form a background for the development and validation effort undertaken by ibstpi.

QUESTIONS FOR CONSIDERATION

Why is it important for a profession, such as that of evaluator, to have a set of standards or guidelines for practice?

Which of the standards and guidelines seem most applicable to you and your organization?

What other standards and guidelines might be used to inform evaluation practice?

CHAPTER

THE VALIDATION RESEARCH

This chapter will enable you to accomplish the following:

■ Describe the ibstpi Evaluator Competencies development and validation processes

■ Describe how the results of this work could be applied to various kinds of evaluators working in different organizational settings and cultures

In Chapter 3, we presented the overall ibstpi approach to competency development. In this chapter, we provide the details on the competency development and validation process for the Evaluator Competencies. We begin by describing the purpose and scope of the study and then turn to the specific procedures and the instrumentation. This is followed by a description of the sample and the results of the validation.

PURPOSE AND SCOPE OF THE STUDY

The final set of standards for evaluators was the product of a global validation research study. This research sought to determine the extent to which the draft of the Evaluator Competencies and their related performance statements reflected the attitudes, skills, and knowledge most critical to individuals who undertake evaluation projects in for-profit and not-for-profit organizations, military organizations, and government agencies evaluating their own internal programs. More specifically, the validation research was designed to establish (1) the level of criticality of each of the competencies and performance statements for practitioners in these settings, (2) that the language used was consistent with that used in the workplace, (3) that it was culturally appropriate outside of North America, and (4) that no critical areas of evaluation practice had been omitted from the standards. The input from the validation feedback was used to accept, modify, or reject the draft competencies and performance statements, thereby producing a final set of standards for evaluators.

PROCEDURES

In this section, we discuss the three phases of the research study. These included a review of the foundational research, competency drafting, and competency validation and rewriting.

■ **Phase I: Review of foundational research.** In undertaking this research study, ibstpi followed the systematic approach laid out elsewhere (Richey, 2002). Initially we undertook an extensive literature search, including a review of academic programs, courses, and training modules in evaluation provided by universities' evaluation curricula in several countries. Simultaneously, we contacted professional associations for evaluators in North America, Australia, and Europe, seeking any listings of competencies or related research as well as training courses and modules offered by these associations.

■ **Phase 2: Competency drafting.** Using these data and the basic premises and assumptions of the previous sets of ibstpi competencies, a subset of the ibstpi Board with particular expertise in evaluation work developed an initial draft set of standards. The next step was to convene an advisory group of recognized evaluation experts and practitioners from North America, Australasia, and Europe who were asked to review the draft standards through two iterations. In addition, 125 practitioners, academics, and a small number of graduate students at three ibstpi workshops in Australia reviewed the draft standards and provided valuable feedback.

▪ **Phase 3: Competency validation and rewriting.** From the expert reviews, we produced a final draft set of standards to be globally validated. This final draft set was reviewed and approved by the entire ibstpi Board.

The instrument based on the final draft set of domains, competencies, and performance statements, along with specific demographic items, was pilot tested. It was then translated into French and Spanish and back-translated into English. The French and Spanish versions were reviewed and revised by native speakers familiar with evaluation. The three versions of the instrument (in English, French, and Spanish) were then administered through the ibstpi web site to evaluation practitioners and academics in diverse geographical locations and work environments.

The results of the validation study were analyzed and reviewed by the subset of the board, and a revised set of standards developed. These were reviewed by the full ibstpi Board and the expert advisory group, who both agreed on these as the final set of standards for evaluators. Reliability for the section of the instrument containing the domains, competencies, and performance was calculated using Cronbach's alpha. This section of the instrument had a high level of reliability with $\alpha = .99$.

Instrumentation

The instrument used in the validation study began with an introduction to the study, indicating its purpose and the use of the data, and provided the informed consent materials approved by the Institutional Review Board of Oregon State University. It then proceeded through three separate sections: the criticality statements, the respondent background characteristics, and additional comments.

Section 1: Criticality Statements The 14 competencies and 86 performance statements were listed, and respondents were asked to assign an importance rating to each in relation to their work role. The rating employed a 5-point Likert scale where 5 represented a very high level of importance in the respondent's work as an evaluator, and 1 represented none. Competencies were shown in a shaded bar, with performance statements sequentially numbered below. Exhibit 7.1 shows the validation survey items for two performance statements related to the competency *Communicate effectively in written, oral, and visual form.*

EXHIBIT 7.1 An Example of the Items in the Validation Survey

Use a scale of 1 to 5 to indicate how important the statement is in relation to your work as an evaluator.

1 = none, 2 = low, 3 = moderate, 4 = high, 5 = very high

Evaluator Competency/ Performance Statement	Level of Importance in My Work
1 Communicate effectively in written, oral, and visual form	1☐ 2☐ 3☐ 4☐ 5☐
1a Use verbal and nonverbal language appropriate to the audience, context, and culture	1☐ 2☐ 3☐ 4☐ 5☐
1b Use active listening skills	1☐ 2☐ 3☐ 4☐ 5☐

Section 2: Respondent Background Characteristics This section contained 12 questions seeking demographic data to establish a rationale for the level of generalizability of data. Questions covered evaluation role, organizational setting, geographical region, educational level and whether evaluation was studied at university, field of occupational expertise, years doing evaluation, percentage of time spent on evaluation, whether respondent was a member of a professional association for evaluators, gender, and age.

Section 3: Additional Comments The survey contained three open-ended questions seeking information on any competencies that should be added or reworded and general feedback.

Sample Selection The ibstpi Board sent out information to more than 40 professional associations for trainers or evaluators around the world, academic programs in evaluation in several countries, listservs and professional networks, conference participants, and the worldwide contacts of ibstpi Board members. Individuals visiting the ibstpi web site were also made aware of the survey and could take it if they wished. Because the sample was not selected on a random or systematic basis, the profile data cannot be assumed to be truly representative of the practitioners for whom these standards have been developed. Nonetheless, there is considerable diversity among the respondents, as is described below.

Demographics of Respondents The sample was a diverse group of 443 respondents, although not all respondents answered all questions. Table 7.1 presents the personal profile of the respondents. In terms of education, the majority possessed a master's level (47 percent) or

TABLE 7.1 **Personal Profile of the Respondents in the ibstpi Evaluator Competency Validation Study (*N* = 443)**

Characteristic	Respondents, No. (%)
Formal education, degree level	
Less than bachelor's	13 (4.2)
Bachelor's	46 (14.8)
Master's	147 (47.3)
Post-master's or doctoral	105 (33.8)
Gender	
Female	168 (55.1)
Male	137 (44.9)
Age, yr	
20–30	26 (8.8)
31–40	63 (21.2)
41–50	83 (27.9)
51–60	99 (33.3)
61+	26 (8.8)

a post-master's or doctoral level (34 percent) degree. Slightly more of the respondents were female (55 percent). The typical respondent was between 41 and 60 years of age (61 percent). This sample appears to be more educated and slightly older than those participating in either the validation research for the ibstpi Training Manager Standards (Foxon, Richey, Roberts, & Spannaus, 2003) or the Instructional Design Standards (Richey, Fields, & Foxon, 2001). This may be because evaluation work is not something that most practitioners do when they begin to work in the training and learning field.

Table 7.2 provides the details on the occupational backgrounds of the respondents. The respondents primarily worked in for-profit organizations

TABLE 7.2 **Occupational Profile of the Respondents in the ibstpi Study (*N* = 443)**

Characteristic	Respondents, No. (%)
Primary organizational settings for work	
Educational institution	58 (20.1)
Association or nonprofit	46 (15.9)
Government agency	33 (11.4)
Manufacturing	23 (8.0)
Health care	18 (6.2)
High-tech	18 (6.2)
Financial services	10 (3.5)
Military	10 (3.5)
Intergovernmental organization	8 (2.8)
Retail sales	8 (2.8)
Telecommunications	7 (2.4)

Transportation	7 (2.4)
Utilities	4 (1.4)
Pharmaceuticals	2 (0.7)
Software development	2 (0.7)
Other	35 (12.1)
Fields of expertise	
Education, including instructional design and adult education	62 (20.3)
Training and development	45 (14.7)
Human resources or organizational development	40 (13.1)
Evaluation	34 (11.1)
Business	23 (7.5)
Management and administration	21 (6.9)
Psychology	17 (5.6)
Communications	11 (3.6)
Science	11 (3.6)
Information systems and computer science	8 (2.6)
Engineering	3 (1.0)
Medicine	2 (0.7)
Other	29 (9.5)

of various types (36 percent), educational institutions (20 percent), and associations or nonprofits (16 percent), with the remainder in government agencies (11 percent) or the military (3 percent). Respondents were asked to nominate their primary areas of expertise and could select a maximum of two. The table shows that respondents have expertise in a wide variety of fields, but the highest percentage (20 percent) nominated education, including instructional design and adult education. The corporate fields where evaluation is most often positioned—training and development or human resources or organizational development—accounted for almost 30 percent, with 15 percent selecting training and development and 13 percent human resources or organizational development. Only 11 percent specifically reported evaluation as their primary field of expertise, suggesting that most of the respondents are not trained in evaluation although, for many, it has become a requirement of their job role.

Table 7.3 displays the profile of the respondents specifically as related to their role as an evaluator. Most of the respondents reported that they functioned as an employee or internal consultant (66 percent) whereas the remainder served as an external consultant to various organizations. The primary regions in which these respondents were

TABLE 7.3 **Evaluator Profile of the Respondents in the ibstpi Study (N = 443)**

Characteristic	Respondents, No. (%)
Evaluator role	
Employee or internal consultant	207 (65.9)
External consultant	107 (34.1)
Primary regions for evaluation work	
United States and Canada	219 (69.3)
Australia and New Zealand	29 (9.2)
Western Europe	20 (6.3)

Asia	19 (6.0)
Eastern Europe	13 (4.1)
Africa and Middle East	9 (2.8)
South America	7 (2.2)
Years in evaluation	
Less than 1	2 (0.6)
1–5	95 (30.4)
6–10	76 (24.3)
11–15	45 (14.4)
16–20	30 (10.0)
More than 20	65 (20.1)
Courses in evaluation during education	
Yes	210 (67.7)
No	100 (32.3)
Membership in an evaluation association	
Yes	150 (48.9)
No	157 (51.1)

located and worked were the United States and Canada (69 percent), Australia and New Zealand (9 percent), Western Europe (6 percent), Asia (6 percent), and Eastern Europe (4 percent), with only a few in Africa and the Middle East (3 percent) or in South America (2 percent).

Although strenuous efforts were made to reach professionals throughout the world, most of the respondents were located in North America. This percentage, however, is much lower than in the ibstpi validation efforts for instructional designers (Richey et al., 2001) or for training managers (Foxon et al., 2003). Many respondents had worked five years or less in evaluation (30 percent), but a surprising number (65 [21 percent]) indicated having worked more than 20 years in the field. Most of the respondents (68 percent) reported that they had taken evaluation courses during their education. Nevertheless, less than half (49 percent) indicated that they were members of an evaluation association.

RATINGS OF CRITICALITY

In the following section, we report the results of the ratings of criticality and importance. We begin with an overview of the ratings and of the domains and then turn to the specific competencies and performance statements.

TABLE 7.4 **Level of Support for the Four Competency Domains by Average Number and Percentage at the Three Highest Levels**

| Competency Domain | Ratings of Competencies Within Domains* | | | |
	4.5–5.0 No. (%)	4.0–4.49 No. (%)	3.5–3.99 No. (%)	Totals Across Competency Domains No. (%)
Professional foundations	2 (40)	2 (40)	1 (20)	5 (100)
Planning and designing the evaluation		2 (67)	1 (33)	3 (100)
Implementing the evaluation		1 (50)	1 (50)	2 (100)
Managing the evaluation		3 (75)	1 (25)	4 (100)

*4.5–5.0 = very high importance, 4.0–4.49 = high importance, and 3.5–3.99 = moderate importance.

General Reactions

Overall, the respondents supported the Evaluator Competencies at a high level by assigning high criticality ratings to most of the items, using a 5-point importance scale (5 indicating "very high"; 4, "high"; 3, "moderate"; 2, "low"; and 1, "none").

Table 7.4 presents the ratings for the four competency domains, showing the number and percentage of competencies within each domain receiving the various averages in ratings. Table 7.5 displays the ratings for the performance statements clustered within the four domains, again indicating the number and percentage of performance statements having certain levels of ratings. The results show that *Professional Foundations* and *Managing the Evaluation* are more highly rated than *Planning and Designing the Evaluation* or *Implementing the Evaluation*.

TABLE 7.5 Level of Support for the Performance Statements Within the Four Domains by Average Number and Percentage at Two of the Highest Levels

| | Ratings of Performance Statements* | | |
| | | | Total Across Competency |
Competency Domain	4.0–4.49 No. (%)	3.5–3.99 No. (%)	Domains No. (%)
Professional foundations	20 (64.5)	11 (35.5)	31 (100)
Planning and designing the evaluation	10 (47.6)	11 (52.4)	21 (100)
Implementing the evaluation	5 (38.5)	8 (61.5)	13 (100)
Managing the evaluation	11 (52.4)	10 (47.6)	21 (100)
Total across competencies	46 (53.5)	40 (46.5)	86 (100)

*See Table 7.4 for description of levels.

A further indication of the level of general support for the competencies appeared in the responses to the open-ended items. Most of the respondents (81 percent) did not indicate any additional competencies. The following are typical of the responses from those who did comment:

- "I think the list encompassed required skills, *all* of which are critical."

- "I found the skills competencies to be very comprehensive."

- "The list was comprehensive and accurate."

COMPETENCY RANKING

Table 7.6 provides more specific results and shows the mean criticality rating and the related variance for each individual competency. The variances across all the competencies appear to be similar. Finally, based on the mean criticality ratings, the competencies are ranked from 1 to 14.

Three of the top five ranked competencies were those within the *Professional Foundations* domain: *Communicate effectively* (ranked number 1), *Observe ethical and legal standards* (number 2), and *Establish and maintain professional credibility* (number 5). The communication competency was also ranked number 1 in the training manager validation study (Foxon et al., 2003) and the instructional design validation study (Richey et al., 2001). The importance of this competency reflects the fact that professionals working in all these areas depend on clear and effective communications to accomplish their work. Furthermore, the high rankings given to observing standards and maintaining credibility indicated that evaluators working within organizational settings rely on their integrity and professional credibility to accomplish much of their work. In addition, because the majority of respondents reside in North America, it may also be a reflection of the increasing concern with ethical practice in organizations following a number of high-profile cases and related government legislation.

The third-ranked competency was *Analyze and interpret data* within the *Managing the Evaluation* domain, and the fourth-ranked competency was *Develop an effective evaluation plan* within the *Planning and Designing the Evaluation* domain. In addition, because there is little difference in rankings between 3 and 4, the results indicate that evaluators see the need for a plan and the analysis or interpretation competencies as equal in importance. The high rankings of these competencies relate

TABLE 7.6 Criticality Ratings of the 2006 ibstpi Evaluator Competencies

Domain	Competency	No.	Mean	SD	Rank
Professional foundations	Communicate effectively in written, oral, and visual form	443	4.63	0.70	1
	Demonstrate awareness of the politics of evaluation	369	3.67	0.98	14
	Demonstrate effective interpersonal skills	401	4.27	0.76	7
	Establish and maintain professional credibility	401	4.36	0.76	5
	Observe ethical and legal standards	443	4.50	0.82	2
Planning and designing the evaluation	Develop an effective evaluation plan	369	4.40	0.84	4
	Develop an evaluation management plan	351	3.97	0.96	11
	Devise data collection strategies to support the evaluation questions and design	351	4.25	0.90	8
Implementing the evaluation	Collect data	337	4.20	0.95	9
	Pilot test the data collection instruments and procedures	337	3.75	0.95	13

(Continued)

Domain	Competency	No.	Mean	SD	Rank
Managing the evaluation	Analyze and interpret data	337	4.42	0.88	3
	Disseminate and follow up the findings and recommendations	329	4.08	0.90	10
	Monitor the evaluation plan	329	3.85	0.98	12
	Work effectively with personnel and stakeholders	329	4.34	0.82	6

specifically to the work of an evaluator and to the heart of evaluation. Certainly, analyzing and interpreting data represent a critical competency for most evaluators because the work involves making sense of data for a client or organization.

The competency labeled *Disseminate and follow up the findings and recommendations* received a criticality rating of only 4.08 and was tenth in the ranking. This is surprising given the extensive interest among professional evaluators in the area of evaluation use. What it may reflect is that those undertaking evaluations within organizations are focusing their attention on the planning and conduct of the evaluation because those are areas under an evaluator's direct control. Issues related to dissemination and follow up of the findings and recommendations are assumed to be under the purview of the decision maker. As Torres, Preskill, and Piontek (2005) argue, dissemination involves more than simply writing a final report, and the savvy evaluator will identify creative, and not necessarily expensive, means to communicate and disseminate information about the evaluation.

Two competencies received somewhat low ratings: *Pilot test the data collection instruments and procedures* (rated 3.75, ranked 13th) and *Demonstrate awareness of the politics of evaluation* (rated 3.67, ranked 14th). The first of these, related to pilot testing, may indicate that evaluators in organizations are under time and resource pressures, and so this important step gets skipped, as does the needs assessment step in instructional design. Furthermore, it suggests that the respondents are either not aware of the need or knowledgeable about how to do a pilot test. The second competency, that involving politics, may reflect some misconceptions regarding the politics surrounding all evaluations. These issues are discussed in greater detail in Chapter 4. The results from both of these competencies suggest that ibstpi focuses on developing a set of competencies reflecting not only what is but what should be. For this reason, these two competencies emphasizing the criticality of pilot testing and an awareness of political issues within an organization continue to be included in the ibstpi standards despite the criticality rating on the validation study being low.

FACTORS CONTRIBUTING TO SIGNIFICANT DIFFERENCES

In the following sections, we describe some of the differences that emerged when comparing results for specific subgroups. This discussion is based on the findings, and we report only statistically significant results.

Geographic Location

In general, respondents in North America rated competencies more highly than did respondents from other regions of the world. Two competencies, however, showed significant differences in both the ratings and rankings: *Collect data* and *Analyze and interpret data*. In both cases, the North American respondents rated and ranked these competencies significantly higher than did respondents from other regions. There are two possible reasons for this difference. The first is that the respondents in other regions, as compared with those in North America, are able to rely on others to undertake the data collection and analysis work. A second reason may be the increasing focus on randomized designs and higher-level statistics within North America.

Internal or External Evaluator

Evaluators working as employees or internal consultants tended to rate the competencies lower overall than did those who reported working as external consultants. Nevertheless, the rankings of the competencies appeared to be similar for the two groups, with the exception of two competencies. The competency *Establish and maintain professional credibility* received a higher ranking among those working as employees or internal consultants. This may be because the external consultant tends to be endowed with some recognition and credibility; otherwise, they would not have been asked to consult. At the same time, the competency *Devise data collection strategies to support the evaluation questions and design* received a higher ranking among those working as external evaluators. Again, this result may have arisen because devising such data collection strategies is one of the important tasks that tend to be outsourced to external consultants.

Organization Type

Although the respondents came from a variety of types of organizations, an analysis was undertaken by merging these into three main types: (1) government, military, and nonprofit organizations; (2) educational institutions; and (3) for-profit organizations. Only one competency showed significant differences among the respondents from these three types of organizations: *Demonstrate awareness of the politics of evaluation*. In this case, respondents from educational institutions and government, military, and nonprofit organizations rated this competency significantly higher than did those in for-profit organizations. There are three possible reasons for these results. First, it may be that those in for-profit organizations view the politics of evaluation to be related to some political system or governmental action. Second, because many of the evaluators in educational institutions are acting as external evaluators, they may be more aware that they need to understand the politics within each organizational setting. Finally, politics may be less of an issue for those working within organizations that are constantly struggling with limited finances and staff, because more of their energy is being devoted to survival and carrying out their mission.

Years of Experience and Evaluation Association Involvement

Overall, those with more years of experience in evaluation—that is, more than five years—compared with those having fewer years of experience tended to provide higher ratings of all of the competencies. Similarly, respondents indicating some involvement and membership with an evaluation association tended to provide higher ratings than those lacking such involvement. Two specific competencies showed significant differences based on years of experience and involvement with evaluation: *Develop an effective evaluation plan* and *Devise data collection strategies to support the evaluation questions and design.* It may be that respondents with greater evaluation experience recognize the benefits of these evaluation planning activities.

IMPLICATIONS FOR THE FINAL EVALUATOR COMPETENCIES

The validation research, in general, confirmed the ibstpi Evaluator Competencies and Performance Statements as presented in the survey. This was also confirmed by the numerous written comments supporting the competencies and performance statements.

Some of the respondents' written comments did, however, provide a basis for some minor editing of two competencies and 15 performance statements. In addition, two performance statements were eliminated by merging them with other performance statements. One of these involved merging internal and professional networks because the distinction was not relevant (resulting performance statement within competency *3: Establish and maintain effective working relationships*). The other (resulting statement within competency *8: Develop a data collection plan, including protocols and procedures*) merged the development of data collection protocols with the development of the data collection plan, which reflects what is typically done.

There was, however, one area of concern raised by several of the respondents. That concern involved the importance of various approaches and tools specifically used by evaluators. The following are some examples:

- Testing (3 respondents)
- Statistical analyses (2 respondents)
- Use of participatory methods (2 respondents)
- Cost analyses
- *Connaissance des différents outils méthodologiques* [knowledge on different methodological tools]

In addition to a focus on specific evaluation tools, several respondents recognized that for evaluations that take place within organizational settings evaluators need to be familiar with the tools and approaches used by these organizations. The following illustrate some of these comments:

- Ability to quantify behavior or role data with regard to operating and financial numbers (business or financial savvy)

- Ability to apply basic economics to evaluation

- Business acumen, including financial analysis

- *Evaluación financiera, evaluación económica, economía en general* [financial evaluation, economic evaluation, economics in general].

Related to concerns about financial analyses, a few respondents mentioned the importance of systems theory, particularly within an organizational context. Some of these comments follow:

- Ability to apply systems theory-related types of modeling, including systems dynamics, to evaluation.

- Ability to identify components of highly complex organizational systems and to analyze authoritative and persuasive (without authority) relationships among components.

In reviewing these comments and determining the most appropriate action to take, the team was guided by past practice in the validation of draft standards. The ibstpi standards are written for the practitioner population functioning in many different settings, with many different types of stakeholders, and are intended to provide a general but sufficiently detailed guide to practice. The standards cannot incorporate this level of recommended specificity and remain accessible and useful. Nevertheless, given the level of concern raised by the various comments, the ibstpi Board decided to undertake a separate survey to identify the importance of various evaluation approaches and measurement and business tools. The procedures and the results of this work are described in Appendix C.

One other area of concern mentioned by a few of the respondents involved the cross-cultural nature of evaluation work within global organizations today. The following provide some examples:

- Awareness in cultural differences was addressed briefly. With the growth of multicultural organizations, this becomes a more and more important competency for evaluators.

- Competency in language and cultural sensitivity for cross-cultural and cross-national evaluations.

▪ Cultural competence and culturally responsive quantitative, qualitative, and mixed-methods theories of use.

▪ Dealing with nondominant groups: groups of different culture, ethnicity, resource, or needs.

Given that most of the respondents reported working within a single cultural context, at least currently, the board decided that including such a statement was not critical at the present time. In addition, cultural issues are addressed in a general way within the *Professional Foundations* domain. For a particular evaluator or any specific organization, however, the issue of language and cultural competence may be critical and should be examined within the context of each evaluation effort.

CONCLUSIONS

In summary, the validation research work was an integral part of the competency development process. The final list of Evaluator Competencies and Performance Statements was based on the results of this validation research, which included an examination of the broader foundation of empirical research as described in Chapters 2 and 6. The validation effort helped to confirm that the ibstpi Evaluator Competency model was indeed applicable to evaluators working in a variety of organizational settings and national and organizational cultures.

QUESTIONS FOR CONSIDERATION

To what extent does the sample appear to reflect your experiences with other evaluators? What surprises you about the sample?

To what extent do the rankings and ratings seem appropriate to you and your own experience?

Which of the reported differences seem reasonable to you? Which seem somewhat surprising, and why?

CHAPTER

8

FUTURE DIRECTIONS

This chapter will enable you to accomplish the following:

- Identify some areas of future focus for evaluation
- Describe the outsourcing of evaluation
- Discuss the emphasis on professionalism and accountability in evaluation
- Describe the globalization of evaluation

Evaluation is action-driven. It is organized around dynamic yet structured processes for providing people within organizations with the information they need to make critical decisions about the programs or processes in which people participate or about the products with which they are affiliated or by which they are affected. It is a field built around responsiveness, flexibility, and options and unfettered by economic, geographic, social, or cultural boundaries (Bamberger, Rugh, & Mabry, 2006). Although *context* indeed plays a role in how programs, processes, and products unfold, their reach or pervasiveness, and the goals or outcomes that underlie them, the issues decision-makers face in determining their performance, impact, cost-effectiveness, and even appropriateness are quite similar.

The ibstpi Evaluator Competencies reveal much about the practice of evaluation within organizational settings and about those actively engaged in it. The four-domain set collectively depicts practitioners who communicate effectively, value credibility, conduct themselves ethically and responsibly, are politically astute, make data-based decisions informed by personal insight, and use time wisely—their own and others'.

In this chapter, we describe some future directions for evaluators and evaluations within organizational settings. These organizational settings include for-profit organizations and nonprofit organizations and agencies as well as governmental and military organizations focused on their own internal programs, processes, and products. Specifically, we discuss three major trends or directions for such evaluation: outsourcing of evaluation functions, professionalism and accountability, and globalization of evaluation. Furthermore, within each of these trends, the sections outline some possible directions for future work on the Evaluator Competencies.

FOCUS OF EVALUATIONS

Measurement, assessment, and evaluation, particularly focused on internal programs and processes, are gaining importance within organizations. Some argue for the importance of measuring more than profit and loss and suggest that organizations develop a "dashboard" of measures. As with an automobile whose wise owner does not just monitor the gas gauge, an organization, too, should not simply be measured based on profits. Rather, a dashboard of measures, including employee satisfaction, production time, customer satisfaction, as well as profits and losses, need to be gathered, analyzed, and interpreted on an ongoing basis. Currently in many different organizations, human resources (HR) personnel monitor such dashboard measures. Such efforts, however, call for some guidance in these measurement efforts by evaluators functioning within organizational settings, and these evaluators will need to determine the most appropriate and cost-effective methods for measuring and interpreting such organizational data. Future competencies may place increasing emphasis on such organizational measurement issues.

At the same time, more and more emphasis is being placed on determining the return on investment (ROI) of various programs and processes. Furthermore, senior management expects HR and human resources development (HRD) staff to be able to gather and present such data. But this type of evaluation is both difficult and expensive to conduct, and the results may not yield credible information for decision makers. The question, then, becomes whether the time, energy, and money to undertake such an evaluation are worth the cost. In the future, evaluators working within such a setting may need to be able to argue the merits of various approaches to determining ROI and to suggest the most appropriate methods for aiding decision makers.

While concerns with dashboards and ROI proliferate in the organizational world, the evaluation profession has been experiencing methodological growth. Several prominent researchers or practitioners have proposed a dizzying array of strategies, frameworks, techniques, and models. (See Appendix C for a listing of the various tools and techniques included in the special survey.) Unfortunately, these strategies, frameworks, techniques, and models rarely appear or are used in organizational settings; either the person tasked with undertaking the evaluation is unfamiliar with the various options, or the clients and stakeholders cannot be convinced that such approaches will yield needed information. In the future, evaluators working within organizational settings must be able to present some of the new approaches and describe their benefits to decision makers and decision-making.

Technological advances have resulted in a variety of changes to the methods and procedures used by evaluators working within organizational settings. First, the Internet and organizational intranets have enabled surveys to be mounted with ease and data to be gathered from many people in many locations. Second, the data that are gathered—whether through such surveys or other means—can be more easily analyzed and presented in graphic and tabular form. But the ease of data collection and analysis may mask the difficulties that evaluators still encounter when deciding what data should be collected, how such data should be analyzed, and what interpretations should be made of the results. As a result of the technological advances, future evaluators will need not only to be familiar with the various technologies but to further develop their skills in interpreting the results for stakeholders. After all, it is only through the interpretation that the evaluator can influence decision-making.

OUTSOURCING EVALUATION

Major organizations in the United States and Europe downsized their training and development and HRD staffs in the early years of this decade as a result of an economic downturn. Although these organizations are experiencing growth and expansion, they show no signs of rehiring such specialists. Consequently, few major organizations will have one or more internal staff devoted to and competent in evaluation work. Currently this work tends to fall to those in training, HR, or leadership development. It is unlikely that this will change, thus necessitating a deepening of evaluation skill among these practitioners. Such a future direction will make the ibspti standards even more valuable to managers and others in these organizations for selecting and developing the needed competencies to do the work.

With the increasing importance of measurement, assessment, and evaluation within organizations, along with the decrease in knowledgeable and skilled internal personnel, much of this work, particularly the more complex evaluations, will be outsourced to small consulting companies. A major question is whether such consultants will possess relevant training and competencies to undertake these efforts. Alternatively, it may be that these consultants will possess little formal training in evaluation, similar to the outsourcing of e-learning to consultants who often know relatively little about instructional systems design and learning theory. If that future trend holds, the ibstpi standards may prove helpful to organizations when attempting to hire the appropriate expertise for their measurement, assessment, and evaluation projects.

PROFESSIONALISM AND ACCOUNTABILITY

Another trend that may be viewed as in opposition to some of the above statements involves an increasing emphasis on professionalism and accountability within the evaluation community. This trend stems mostly from the work of various evaluation associations throughout the world. To what extent and in what ways this trend might influence evaluators working within organizational setting is not yet completely clear. In this following section, we begin with some definitions of professionalism and accountability and then describe some of the forces emphasizing such professionalism and accountability.

A *profession* is "any type of work which needs special training or a particular skill, often one which is respected because it involves a high level of education" (Cambridge University Press, 2007 n.p.). The ibstpi set of evaluator domains, competencies, and associated performance statements detailed in this book help to substantiate the work of an evaluator in an organizational setting as representing a profession. On a more practical level, these standards inform professional development efforts of which practicing evaluators might avail themselves—whether offered by the organizations for which they work or by associations or institutions that specialize in certification programs or academic credit.

By definition, *professionalism* relates to the conduct of people affiliated with a profession, specifically, their behavior and the ethical code or mores that underlie it, the rules or procedures by which novices become members, and the ways in which they interact and connect with others (McDavid & Hawthorn, 2006). Also core to professionalism is the idea of *accountability,* and the evaluation competencies showcased in this text play an important role in defining and measuring it—whether *personal* or *organizational.*

What is accountability? Dictionaries provide definitions of varying detail; what they share is an emphasis on individual behavior or action. Thus, an accountable individual is "answerable, required to give account (as of one's actions or the discharge of a duty or trust)" (see *American Heritage Dictionary of the English Language* at http:// www.bartleby.com). The person, then, is "responsible or trustworthy, able to defend one's conduct and obligations" (see Dictionary .com at http://dictionary.reference.com/browse/accountable). Common among the varying meanings—and intimately familiar to workplace professionals—is the notion of an obligation to answer to an authority that may impose a penalty for failure.

Within the evaluation profession, there appears to be an increasing emphasis on the development of standards and principles of conduct, many of which were described in Chapters 2 and 6. Such standards and guidelines can be used either formally or informally. Some evaluators, for example, have argued that there should be certification for evaluators, similar to that experienced by certified public accountants. In this case, such standards and guidelines would need to be followed to avoid some penalty. Currently, some training and development associations, like the American Society for Training and Development (ASTD), are putting increasing emphasis on evaluation. (See http://www.astd.org/ astd/Publications/competency_study.htm for details about its certified professional in learning and performance. This is a competency-based certification that clearly marks evaluation as a key competency for training and development and HR practitioners.) Others prefer to use the standards and guidelines as aspirational. Accountability in this case would rest with the individual rather than the organization or association. Depending on the outcome of this argument, future ibstpi Evaluator Competencies may need to take into account the certification and accountability requirements needed by evaluators.

GLOBAL COMPETENCE

In 2003, Scriven proposed a "transdisciplinary" vision of evaluation. He argued that evaluation is versatile, providing "services" (tools such as logic, design, and statistics; techniques; strategies) to *all* disciplines, while "retaining an autonomous structure and research effort of [its] own" (p. 19). Donaldson and Christie (2006) argue, for example, that "evaluation science [enhances] psychology by sorting out which psychological principles and findings are effective for preventing or ameliorating human problems in real-world settings" (p. 248). A clear manifestation of the transdisciplinary view is the sheer number of evaluation journals—*New Directions for Evaluation, Evaluation Practice, Evaluation Quarterly, Evaluation and Change, Evaluation Review,* and *Evaluation and Program Planning*—that cross traditional disciplinary lines, with articles focused on educational settings, government agencies, nonprofit organizations, health care concerns, mental health issues, business and industry settings, and the work of foundations. In addition to the evaluation journals, other journals related to HR, HRD, and performance improvement are publishing articles or issues related to evaluation: *Advances in Developing Human Resources, Human Resource Development Quarterly, Performance Improvement Quarterly, T&D,* and *Training.*

The notion of evaluation as a transdiscipline also helps to explain its growth as a field and a profession—in particular, its *internationalization* (Fitzpatrick, Sanders, & Worthen, 2004). Today, there are more than 75 evaluation societies around the world, many in developing countries. The International Organization for Cooperation in Evaluation (http://ioce.net), formed in 2003, is a "loose alliance of regional and national organizations (associations, societies, networks from around that world" (see http://ioce.net/overview/general.shtml) with a number of specific goals, to wit: building evaluation leadership and evaluation capacity in developing countries; helping practitioners take a more worldly approach to the issues, problems, and questions they investigate; and fostering global collaboration, information sharing, and theory building. The International Development Evaluation Association (http://www.ideas-int.org) focuses more exclusively on *development evaluation* and ways evaluation practice can help to reduce poverty, remove the social and structural constraints that thwart economic and human development, and improve program or project management through transparent decision-making and other inclusive practices (http://www.ideas-int.org/ Profile.aspx).

Globalization of business and industry and of both nonprofit and foundation work also contributes to the globalization of evaluation efforts. Indeed, several respondents in the ibstpi Evaluator Competencies validation survey suggested the importance of cultural and multicultural awareness. For evaluators practicing within such global environments, there will be a need for cultural training and development. Otherwise, such evaluators may be ill prepared for the methodological challenges they face in access to data, for example, or the political, institutional, and organizational settings in which they find themselves. Although the ibstpi Evaluator Competencies appear relevant to cultures and evaluators throughout the world, future evaluators may need more in-depth multicultural and cross-cultural competencies.

CONCLUSIONS

The ibstpi Evaluator Competencies provide a road map for evaluators functioning in today's organizational settings, particularly those undertaking evaluations within government agencies, the military, nonprofit organizations, and business and industry. They also speak to the deepening interest in evaluation within organizations and the anticipated competencies that practitioners in training, learning, and HRD will require in the near future as evaluation and measurement assume greater importance. The standards are future-focused as well, in particular, emphasizing issues that are of less concern, such as the importance of pilot testing to ensure high-quality data and of gaining an awareness of the political nature of each evaluation effort. The use of these standards can help to inform the practice of evaluation and the development of evaluators working within these settings.

QUESTIONS FOR CONSIDERATION

How might these future trends impact the evaluation profession or how evaluations are conducted?

What concerns you (or your colleagues) about some of the emerging ideas, theories, or practices described in this chapter?

What other trends do you see on the horizon? What might be the impact of these trends?

APPENDIX

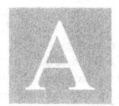

ibstpi AND ITS HISTORY

The International Board of Standards for Training, Performance, and Instruction (ibstpi) is a not-for-profit organization that provides leadership to the human learning and performance communities by setting standards. Its mission is to develop, validate, and promote implementation of international standards to advance training, instruction, learning, and performance improvement for individuals and organizations.

ibstpi grew from the Joint Certification Task Force, which was established in 1977 and sponsored by the Association for Educational Communications and Technology (AECT) and the National Society for Performance and Instruction (now the International Society for Performance Improvement [ISPI]). The Joint Task Force, composed of more than 30 practitioners and academics with expertise in training, performance, and instruction, developed a set of competencies for the instructional designers, published an index linking current publications to competencies, and created prototype assessment procedures. The members of the task force also published articles on professional competence and certification and spoke at professional meetings.

In 1983, to avoid conflict of interest with its parent organizations, the task force reorganized itself as the ibstpi Board. Based on efforts initiated by the task force, the board furthered research and development activities on competencies leading to the publication of competency models. Among these models are the 1986 ibstpi Instructional Design Competencies and Performance Statements, the 1989 ibstpi Training Manager Competencies and Performance Statements, and the 1993 ibstpi

Instructor Competencies. The latter set of competencies is the foundation for many instructor training programs and until September 2003 was the basis of the Certified Technical Trainer certification administered by the Computer Technology Industry Association (ComTIA). More than 3,500 technical instructors have gained certification as Certified Technical Trainers (CTT+) based on the ibstpi standards.

The board acknowledges that changes in the economy, as well as the ongoing development of technology, have an impact on the profession, and it periodically reviews and revises the competency models. This effort has resulted in an updated set of competencies for instructional designers and training managers and for instructors addressing the competencies for online, blended, and face-to-face settings. The latest competency model developed by ibstpi is the Evaluator Competencies (2006) presented in this book. Current projects relate to competencies for online learning and the development of professional certifications associated with the standards.

ibstpi also examines and evaluates training programs and their associated content to provide a designation known as "Recognized ibstpi Materials" (RiM) to approved training programs that have been based on the ibstpi standards.

Currently, the ibstpi Board comprises 15 directors representing the communities they serve, including universities, government departments, businesses, and consultancy practice. Each board member serves as an exemplar of professional practice and the ethics of the profession. In addition, the board consults with advisors, corporate partners, and former board members who contribute to ibstpi's mission.

In recent years, the board has expanded its focus on the international aspect of its name and mission, with directors from Europe, Canada, Japan, and Australia as well as members from the United States. ibstpi places a special interest in globally validating the competencies, and some of the competencies have been translated into other languages. The board meets monthly by conference call and three times a year in various locations around the world. These gatherings are often tied in with conferences and workshops that attract researchers, invited speakers, and participants around a particular theme. In 1998, a conference was held at the University of Bergen in Norway to examine the intersection of instructional design and performance improvement. The following year, the board convened a workshop at Estes Park, Colorado, to consider revisions to the Training Manager competencies. In 2000, ibstpi and

Lancaster University in the United Kingdom jointly sponsored a conference addressing issues of online training delivery. This initiative resulted in the revised instructor competencies. In 2005, ibstpi offered a series of workshops in Australia at the universities in Brisbane, Melbourne, and Sydney on the theme of competencies for instructional designers, instructors, online learners, and evaluators. Comments gathered in those workshops were used in the development of the competencies presented in this book.

APPENDIX

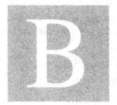

GLOSSARY

Active listening. Paying close attention to what another person is communicating, including the unspoken messages, and reflecting back what has been understood.

Anonymity. Pertains to protecting the identity of respondents or interviewees in an evaluation by ensuring their data cannot be traced back to them.

Benchmark. The industry standard for whatever practice, process, or product is being studied. Related term: Best practice.

Benefit-cost ratio (BCR). See Cost–benefit analysis.

Best practice. A technique or method that is regarded as exemplary on the basis of experience or research. Related term: Benchmark.

Certification. The process used by a professional association or organization to attest that an individual has a specified degree of competence or meets a certain performance standard.

Code of ethics. A set of principles intended to aid members of the field individually and collectively in maintaining a high level of professional conduct (Seels & Richey, 1994). Related term: Ethical standards.

Competence. The state of being well qualified for a task, role, or profession.

Competencies. A set of related knowledge, skills, and attitudes that enables an individual to effectively perform the activities of a given occupation or job function to the standards expected in employment.

Competency modeling. The process resulting in an organized set of competencies and performance indicators.

Confidentiality. The keeping of data or information from unauthorized persons or processes in order to protect the identity of the individual who disclosed it.

Conflict of interest. A situation in which personal business affairs may materially or adversely affect one's relationship with an organization.

Consultant. An individual or organization retained to work on a project because of specific expertise; consultants may be internal or external. Related term: Contractor.

Cost-benefit analysis. A comparison of the economic benefits of the program with the actual and opportunity costs of the program. Related terms: Benefit-cost ratio, trade-off analysis.

Cost-effective. When the value derived from a transaction meets or exceeds the cost of that transaction to an individual or organization.

Cross-cultural. Dealing with or comparing two or more cultures. Related term: intercultural.

Culture. The knowledge, values, and practices shared by a group.

Customer. An organization or person for whom a service is performed; may be internal or external to the organization. Related term: client.

Dashboard. A set of metrics used to provide a quick assessment of a project or process status, presented in a way that is easy to read. The name refers to the fact that it can sometimes look like the dashboard of a car.

Deliverable. A work product that must be completed and delivered as agreed on with a client or sponsor.

Dichotomous. Divided into two distinguished parts or categories.

Digital technologies. Electronic tools that are dependent on computers in some form. Examples used by evaluators include data analysis software, project management software, videoconferencing for interviews, and the like.

Domain. A cluster of related competencies.

Empirical data. Data that come from observation, experiment, or practical experience.

Ethical standards. See Code of ethics.

Evaluation. The systematic collection of information about the characteristics, activities, and outcomes of programs, processes, and products in order to make judgments and decisions about needed improvement or future planning (adapted from Patton, 1997).

Evaluation: Formative. Gathering data on the adequacy of an intervention, process, or product and using this information as a basis for improvement or further development.

Evaluation plan. A set of procedures that will be used to gather evaluation data or related information.

Evaluation strategy. A process for focusing objectives and allocating resources to achieve evaluation goals.

Evaluation: Summative. The systematic gathering of data on the adequacy and outcomes of an intervention, process, or product and using this information for reporting or decision-making purposes.

Evaluator. The person who develops the evaluation plan and conducts the evaluation.

Experienced evaluator. A person with a foundation of formal training in the field, substantial work experience, and the ability to conduct evaluations in various contexts and using a variety of methods.

Expertise. The level of knowledge and experience demonstrated by evaluators who are typically categorized as either novice or experienced.

External evaluator. An evaluator who is not an employee of the organization where the evaluation is taking place. Related terms: Internal evaluator, Consultant.

Field notes. A documented record of observations, interactions, conversations, situational details, and thoughts during the evaluation.

Focus group. A group of people who meet with an evaluator to provide insights, ideas, and observations on a topic related to the evaluation.

Fundamental research skills. Skills that are basic to scientific investigation, including the design of exploratory studies and field tests, instrument design and data collection techniques, and the interpretation and analysis of qualitative and quantitative data.

Gantt chart. A bar chart showing tasks and deadlines necessary for completing a project.

Generic model. A general model, one that is not applicable to a specific situation only.

Human capital metrics. Metrics or measures that relate to human resources, as opposed to plant, equipment, or technological resources.

Intellectual property. The knowledge, processes, and capabilities that a company or an individual has developed; typically protected by copyright.

Internal evaluator. An evaluator employed by the organization where the evaluation is taking place. Related terms: External evaluator, Consultant.

Inter-rater reliability. The degree to which the assessment of a task or performance by two or more raters will yield identical ratings.

Legal standards. The principles and regulations legally governing conduct and established by local, state, or national governments.

Likert scale. A scale with item responses on a continuum, ranging from positive to negative and containing response categories such as "strongly agree," "agree," "not sure," "disagree," and "strongly disagree." The scale generally has between 5 and 7 response categories. Related term: Likert-type survey.

Logic model. A tool that visually describes the chain of events linking program goals, activities, and expected outcomes.

Management plan. A plan for managing the project, setting out the goals and the approaches to be used, and including details about personnel, resources, budgets, time line, and deliverables.

Meta-analysis. A statistical analysis of the data and summary of results from several studies.

Metaevaluation. The evaluation of other evaluations.

Metrics. Measures to indicate progress or achievement, usually in relation to performance, process efficiency, products, services, training, and productivity.

Needs assessment. A systematic process for determining goals, identifying discrepancies between optimal and actual performance, and establishing priorities for action (Briggs, 1977). Related term: needs analysis.

Novice evaluator. A practitioner with little or no formal training and with experience in basic evaluation only.

Outsource. Seek products or vendors outside the organization rather than develop or provide the services from within. Related term: build versus buy.

Performance statement. A detailed explanation of activities that makes up a competency statement.

PERT chart. Program Evaluation Review Technique; PERT charts identify the "critical chain" or the longest path through a project.

Pilot test. A preliminary, small-scale test of evaluation activities to try out procedures or techniques and make any needed adjustments. Related term: usability test.

Practice-oriented atheoretical approach. An approach unrelated to or not based on a theory and focused on what is done in practice.

Professional activities. Conduct that enhances the skill, knowledge, or capacity of a practitioner, including attending professional association meetings and conferences, reading relevant texts, or networking with other practitioners.

Professional credibility. The quality of being trustworthy and believable within one's professional setting.

Professional foundations. Those competencies considered foundational to the field; the base competencies that underpin the field.

Proposal. A document setting out how an evaluator intends to undertake the evaluation and typically including information on time line, resources needed, deliverables, and costs.

Proprietary rights. Information that has value to a company and that is not public knowledge. Related terms: Intellectual property; copyright.

Protocol. A detailed plan or set of procedures for collecting data. An interview protocol will specify how the interview should be conducted and the questions to be asked, for example.

Qualitative data. Information drawn from empirical methods such as case study, interview, focus group, or observation of subjects in their environment. The data cannot be reduced to numerical measurements or subjected to statistical procedures.

Quantitative data. Information that can be expressed in numerical terms, counted, or compared on a scale and represented by statistical scores. Related term: statistical data.

Rating scale. A measurement device in which a respondent must choose a response from choices arranged in a continuum, such as from low to high or good to bad.

Reliability. The degree to which items or instruments consistently yield the same or comparable results.

Response bias. The tendency to favor a certain response over others.

Return on investment. An actual value developed by comparing program costs with benefits to an organization (Phillips, 1997a). Related term: ROI.

Sample. A portion or small segment of the population being studied.

Sampling plan. A document that specifies the procedures for selecting a small but representative group (i.e., a sample) from the population being studied. Related term: sampling procedures.

Self-report. A data collection method in which the evaluator asks those being evaluated to report on their own behavior, rather than using a more objective method to gather data.

Stakeholder. Someone with a vested interest in the project outcomes, including, for example, a program developer, learner, manager, third party, team member, colleague, and customer. Related term: sponsor.

Standards. Statements of expectations of performance or levels of knowledge in a specific content domain or job role.

Taxonomy. The classification of data into a hierarchy to indicate their relationships.

Test item. A question on a test. Related term: survey item.

Threats to trustworthiness. Conditions or practices that detract from the reliability and validity of data.

Training. Learning that is provided to improve workplace performance.

Transfer. The application of knowledge and skills acquired in an instructional setting to another environment, typically a work setting.

Triangulation. The comparison of results from three or more data sources or other data methods to establish the accuracy of the findings.

Validation. The process of determining the extent to which competencies and performance statements are supported by the profession.

Validity. The degree to which items measure what they are intended to measure. Related term: valid test items.

APPENDIX

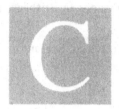

EVALUATION TOOLS
AND APPROACHES

As described in Chapter 7 on the validation research, a common recommendation from survey respondents concerned specific evaluation tools and approaches. That level of detail was not appropriate for the validation of evaluator competencies, but the evaluation team recognized the need to determine the importance of these as background information for evaluators and those interested in evaluator competencies. This appendix contains details of a special survey that was undertaken to gather this information.

PROCEDURES

A comprehensive listing of evaluation tools and approaches was developed. The resulting survey instrument and procedures were reviewed and approved by the Oregon State University Institutional Review Board. Respondents were asked to indicate the level of importance of each tool in their evaluation practice (very high importance, high importance, moderate importance, low importance, or no importance). The tool was administered to groups of evaluators participating in the following conferences or workshops:

- Academy of Human Resource Development conference in Indianapolis

- American Evaluation Association conference in Portland, Oregon

- ibstpi-sponsored workshops in Brisbane, Melbourne, and Sydney, Australia

- HRD Across Europe (Oxford, England)

RESULTS

The results will list the evaluation tools and approaches according to their order of rated importance.

Evaluation Tools and Approaches

(5 = Very High Importance, 4 = High Importance, 3 = Moderate Importance, 2 = Low Importance, 1 = No Importance)

Evaluation Tools and Approaches	Mean	Standard Deviation	Respondents
Needs assessment	4.77	1.19	30
Individual interviews	4.68	0.54	31
Questionnaire and survey design	4.53	0.82	30
Formative evaluation	4.37	0.89	30
Participatory methods	4.27	0.74	30
Summative evaluation	4.23	0.84	31
Process evaluation	4.19	0.79	31
Case study methods	4.13	0.92	31
Focus groups	4.10	0.98	29
Level 3 evaluation	4.07	1.11	27
Process mapping	3.96	0.98	28
Behavioral observations	3.90	1.08	29
Level 2 evaluation	3.89	1.22	27

Evaluation Tools and Approaches	Mean	Standard Deviation	Respondents
Critical incident method	3.88	1.03	24
Testimonials	3.79	1.07	28
Theory-driven evaluation	3.78	0.97	28
Impact mapping	3.75	1.16	20
Success case method	3.73	0.96	26
Level 1 evaluation	3.70	1.41	27
Logic models	3.68	1.25	25
Level 4 evaluation	3.67	1.33	27
Return-on-investment (ROI)	3.66	1.26	29
Systems theory	3.63	1.04	28
Cost analysis	3.57	1.22	30
Cost-benefit analysis	3.57	1.27	30
Open systems approach	3.56	1.00	25
Development evaluation	3.55	1.26	22
Cost-effectiveness analysis	3.50	1.32	28
Parametric statistics	3.48	1.19	25
Behavioral event interviewing	3.46	0.93	24
Quasi-experimental designs	3.45	1.18	29
Psychometrics	3.44	1.18	28
Reactionnaires	3.33	0.86	21
Appreciative inquiry	3.29	1.22	24
Non-parametric statistics	3.25	1.19	24
Evaluability assessment	3.17	1.37	23
Constructivist evaluation	3.05	1.39	20
Experimental designs	3.03	1.25	30
Ethnography	2.96	1.24	25
Demand analysis	2.94	1.48	17
Item-response theory	2.87	1.06	23
Phenomenology	2.86	1.25	22
Confirmative evaluation	2.53	1.02	19
Discounted cash-flow technique	2.45	1.44	22

In addition to the tools rated by each of the respondents, some other tools were mentioned by individual respondents, including 360-degree evaluation; context, input, process, and product evaluations (CIPP); evaluation-specific methodologies; large system/large group evaluation; and online tools and web surveys.

APPENDIX

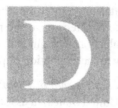

ANNOTATED BIBLIOGRAPHY

The following is a list of books, chapters, articles, and journals that are useful to evaluators, whether novice or experienced. The references are grouped according to the four domains of the ibstpi Evaluator Standards.

PROFESSIONAL FOUNDATIONS

Advances in Developing Human Resources (2005), 7(1).
This journal issue focuses specifically on evaluation in organizational settings and includes articles by Robert Brinkerhoff, Elwood Holton III, Jack Phillips, Darlene Russ-Eft, Hallie Preskill, and Richard Swanson.

American Evaluation Association (2004, July). *Guiding principles for evaluators.* Retrieved March 24, 2007, from http:www.eval.org/Publications/GuidingPrinciples.asp.
These guiding principles were ratified by the membership of the American Evaluation Association. They provide an overview of critical issues to be addressed by evaluators.

American Journal of Evaluation.
One of the journals of the American Evaluation Association. This interdisciplinary journal publishes articles primarily from North America. Each issue also includes an evaluation ethics case study.

Australasian Evaluation Society Inc. (reprint 2006). *Guidelines for the ethical conduct of evaluation.* Australasian Evaluation Society Inc. Retrieved March 25, 2007, from http://www.aes.asn.au.
These guidelines are intended to promote the ethical practice of evaluation and are meant to help evaluators recognize and resolve ethical issues arising in the course of an evaluation. The guidelines focus on the evaluation of programs but also apply to the evaluation of policies and strategies.

Evaluation: The International Journal of Theory, Research and Practice.
Published by Sage in the United States, in association with the Tavistock Institute, United Kingdom. This interdisciplinary journal has articles from Europe, North America, Asia, and Australasia. Available online at http://evi.sagepub.com.

Glossary of key terms in evaluation and results based management (2002). Retrieved March 25, 2007, from http://www.oecd.org/dataoecd/29/21/2754804.pdf.
This provides a multilingual evaluation glossary in English, French, and Spanish. Italian and German versions are also available. OECD [Organisation for Economic Cooperation and Development] Development Assistance Committee, Network on Development Evaluation.

Joint Committee on Standards for Educational Evaluation. *Program evaluation standards.* Retrieved March 24, 2007, from http://www.eval.org/EvaluationDocuments/progeval.html.
These represent standards that are appropriate for all types of evaluators working in a variety of fields and settings. They include standards related to utility, feasibility, propriety, and accuracy.

Nadler, D. A. (2005). Confessions of a trusted counselor. *Harvard Business Review, 83*(9), 68–77.
This article provides some suggestions for working with top executives. Such suggestions can also be applied to working with stakeholders and presenting evaluation results.

New Directions in Program Evaluation.
One of the journals of the American Evaluation Association, published quarterly. Each issue focuses on a particular topic, with an issue editor knowledgeable about that topic.

Practical Assessment, Research, and Evaluation.
This journal provides access to refereed articles about methodological issues, trends, research developments, and practices on evaluation from a variety of settings. Available online at http://pareonline.net.

Preskill, H., & Russ-Eft, D. (2005). *Building evaluation capacity: 72 activities for teaching and training*. Thousand Oaks, Calif.: Sage.
This text includes various activities to introduce evaluations into organizations. These activities can be used with stakeholders to involve them in and increase their knowledge about evaluation.

Russ-Eft, D. (2004). Ethics in a global world: An oxymoron? *Evaluation and Program Planning, 27*, 349–356.
This journal article considers various ethical dilemmas that can surface when undertaking evaluations in different organizational and national cultures. It outlines some of the dilemmas posed by the various ethical standards and guidelines.

Russ-Eft, D. (2004). In search of ethics and integrity. In J. Woodall, M. Lee, & J. McGoldrick (Eds.), *New frontiers in human resource development*, pp. 43–57. London: Routledge.
This chapter examines the use of ethical standards in human resource development and examines some of the approaches to the development of ethical standards and guidelines.

PLANNING AND DESIGNING THE EVALUATION

Barksdale, S., & Lund, T. (2001). *Rapid evaluation*. Alexandria, Va.: American Society for Training and Development.
This book shows how to approach evaluation strategically and link results to organizational goals, strategies, and performance indicators. Included are dozens of evaluation tools, checklists, and examples to help in building a comprehensive evaluation strategy.

Brinkerhoff, R. O. (2003). *The success case method: Find out quickly what's working and what's not*. San Francisco: Berrett-Koehler.
Success case evaluation is a breakthrough technique that is easier, faster, and cheaper than competing approaches and provides compelling evidence that decision makers can actually use. This book takes the reader through the method in simple-to-understand steps.

Brinkerhoff, R. O. (2006). *Telling training's story: Evaluation made simple, credible, and effective*. San Francisco: Berrett-Koehler.
This is the follow-up to Brinkerhoff's 2003 book on success case evaluation and elaborates on the power of that method to evaluate training. It also offers practical step-by-step guidelines for increasing the return on investment of future learning and performance initiatives and

provides case studies from four major companies showing how they used success case evaluation.

Broad, M. L., & Newstrom, J. W. (1992). *Transfer of training: Action-packed strategies to ensure high payoff from training investments.* Reading, Mass.: Addison-Wesley.

The authors present a systematic process for bringing managers and trainees into the transfer process to ensure a much greater payoff from training initiatives. The book contains many practical strategies.

Combs, W. L., & Falletta, S. V. (2000). *The targeted evaluation process.* Alexandria, Va.: American Society for Training and Development.

This text shows how to manage training evaluation with an organized and systematic approach to build flexible interventions, determine whether performance interventions achieved goals, and how to partner with stakeholders throughout the process. Practical tools, templates, and sample questions are included throughout.

Davidson, E. J. (2005). *Evaluation methodology basics: The nuts and bolts of sound evaluation.* Thousand Oaks, Calif.: Sage.

Davidson provides a step-by-step guide to doing an evaluation. She focuses on the big-picture questions and explains how to combine a mix of qualitative and quantitative data to draw conclusions. This book contains useful rubrics and flowcharts that may be used during each stage of an evaluation.

Dessinger, J. C., & Moseley, J. L. (2004). *Confirmative evaluation: Practical strategies for valuing continuous improvement.* San Francisco: Pfeiffer.

This book offers trainers, consultants, evaluation professionals, and human resources practitioners a hands-on resource for understanding and applying the principles of confirmative evaluation—the marriage of evaluation and continuous improvement—to establish the effectiveness, efficiency, impact, and value of the training over time.

Digital resources for evaluators. Compiled by Catherine Callow-Heusser (cheusser@endvision.net). Version: November 2002. Retrieved March 25, 2007, from http://www.resources4evaluators.info/index.htm.

This web site contains numerous links to Internet resources such as communities of evaluators, online discussion groups, companies and consultants, texts and documents, instruments, data, surveys, statistics, software, funding, employment, and education and training in evaluation.

Fitzpatrick, J. L., Sanders, J. R., & Worthen, B. R. (2004). *Program evaluation: Alternative approaches and practical guidelines* (3rd ed.). Boston: Pearson Education.

This book is designed for both novices and experienced evaluators. Evaluation techniques discussed are those of process with a focus on planning and execution. All precepts are illustrated by a running "case," a technique that showcases what happens when stakeholders and participants begin to actively engage in the process.

Gupta, K., Sleezer, C., & Russ-Eft, D. (2007). *A practical guide to needs assessment* (2nd ed.). San Francisco: Pfeiffer and American Society for Training and Development.

This book outlines four designs for undertaking needs assessments, which can be considered a type of evaluation. The four designs include knowledge and skills assessment, job and task analysis, competency-based needs assessment, and strategic needs assessment. It contains templates and tools that can be used or adapted.

Hale, J. (2002). *Performance-based evaluation: Tools and techniques to measure the impact of training.* San Francisco: Jossey-Bass/Pfeiffer.

This book focuses on real-world applications, tips and techniques, tools, and common problems or missteps that evaluators face (or make). Topics covered include productive ways to measure effectiveness, efficiency, hard and soft skills, elective and mandatory training, sampling, and data analysis.

Hilbert, J., Preskill, H., & Russ-Eft, D. (1997). *Evaluating training.* Chap. 5. In L. J. Bassi & D. Russ-Eft (Eds.), *What works: Assessment, development, and measurement.* Alexandria, Va.: American Society for Training and Development.

This very readable chapter reviews four decades of research on training evaluation, providing insights into different ways of evaluating and various models that can be used. The chapter concludes with a list of issues that trainers should consider when undertaking evaluation.

Kirkpatrick, D. L. (Ed.). (1998). *Another look at evaluating training programs.* Alexandria, Va.: American Society for Training and Development.

This is a compilation of articles on evaluation of training programs from the 1990s that provides an overview of theoretical and philosophical approaches to training evaluation as well as specific approaches and techniques for evaluating training. The book also includes sections on creating tests and employee surveys to collect data.

Kirkpatrick, D. L., & Kirkpatrick, J. D. (2005). *Evaluating training programs: The four levels* (3rd ed.). San Francisco: Berrett-Koehler.

D. L. Kirkpatrick's four-level model for evaluating training programs has become the most widely used approach to training evaluation in the corporate, government, and academic worlds. In the third edition of this classic, the Kirkpatricks offer new ideas and procedures for continued quality evaluation of the four levels in today's workplace.

McCain, D. (2005). *Evaluation basics.* Alexandria, Va.: American Society for Training and Development.

This book shows how to connect evaluation to performance, program design, and bottom-line value. It includes a chapter dealing with how biases creep into all levels of evaluation and a chapter on how to communicate evaluation results effectively. Practical examples, worksheets, checklists, tips, and notes are found throughout the book.

Martineau, J., & Hannum, K. (2004). *Evaluating the impact of leadership development: A professional guide.* Greensboro, N.C.: Center for Creative Leadership.

The approach to evaluation presented in this book can be applied in a variety of contexts, but the focus here is on the evaluation of leadership development initiatives. The authors provide 16 evaluation templates that can be used without copyright permission.

Parry, S. B. (2000). *Evaluating the impact of training.* Alexandria, Va.: American Society for Training and Development.

This book's 26 lessons guide evaluators through every step of the evaluation process and illustrate the steps with real-life examples. Helpful tools and checklists are included.

Patton, M. Q. (1997). *Utilization-focused evaluation: The new century text* (3rd ed.). Thousand Oaks, Calif.: Sage.

This book describes how to conduct program evaluations so that they will be useful and used. Each chapter contains a review of the relevant literature and actual case examples to illustrate major points.

Performance Improvement Quarterly (1997). *10*(2). Special issue on transfer of training to transfer of learning.

This special issue includes seven articles on transfer by well-known practitioners in the field, an updated literature review by Kevin Ford, and a selected bibliography.

Phillips, J. J. (1997). *Handbook of training evaluation and measurement methods* (3rd ed.). Houston: Gulf.
This book provides tools for demonstrating the profitability of training and other interventions. It contains case studies and numerous examples and is an excellent reference book.

Phillips, J. J., & Stone, R. D. (2002). *How to measure training results.* Alexandria, Va.: American Society for Training and Development.
This practical book provides guidelines, including reproducible worksheets, to answer such questions as, what did a training program add to the organization's performance and the bottom line? Did it work? If so, why? And if not, what should be done differently?

Robinson, D. G., & Robinson, J. C. (1989). *Training for impact: How to link training to business needs and measure the results.* San Francisco: Jossey-Bass.
This book showcases how evaluation can improve fundamental business practices and behaviors (both individual and collective) when they are purposefully linked to the organizational mission and vision. The authors present evaluation as a core strategic function and not merely an activity to complete in an organization. Useful examples of both tools and analytical strategies are provided.

Rothwell, W. J., & Kazanas, H. C. (2004). Evaluating instruction. In *Mastering the instructional design process: A systematic approach* (3rd ed.). San Francisco: Pfeiffer.
This chapter provides in-depth guidance for practitioners undertaking formative and summative evaluation of instructional programs. Several useful checklists are included.

Russ-Eft, D., & Hoover, A. (2005). The joys and challenges of experimental and quasi-experimental designs. In R. A. Swanson & E. F. Holton III (Eds.), *Research in organizations: Foundations and methods of inquiry.* San Francisco: Berrett-Koehler.
This chapter covers the basic experimental and quasi-experimental designs, presenting potential advantages and challenges. It also provides examples of the designs used within organizational settings.

Russ-Eft, D., & Preskill, H. (2001). *Evaluation in organizations: A systematic approach to enhancing learning, performance, and change.* Cambridge, Mass.: Perseus.
This book is a valuable resource for novice and experienced evaluators, including chapters with detailed discussion of data collection methods,

developing surveys, using focus groups and interviews, dealing with political issues, managing the evaluation project, and reporting evaluation results.

Swanson, R. A., & Holton, E. F. (1999). *Results: How to assess performance, learning, and perceptions in organizations.* San Francisco: Berrett-Koehler.
This practical book provides a five-step assessment process that enables professionals to demonstrate organizational results from training and human resource interventions. Case examples are provided to demonstrate their points.

IMPLEMENTING THE EVALUATION PLAN

Bradburn, N., Sudiman, S., & Wansink, B. (2004). *Asking questions: The definitive guide to questionnaire design—for market research, political polls, and social and health questionnaires.* San Francisco: Jossey-Bass.
This text focuses on the types of questions used in interviews or structured questionnaires and the challenges associated with web-based data gathering, analysis, and reporting. The book is organized into three parts: social context of asking questions, specific techniques for posing questions associated with behaviors and attitudes, and the nuts-and-bolts of survey design, organization, and layout.

Dillman, D. A. (2007). *Mail and internet surveys: The tailored design method.* Hoboken, N.J.: Wiley.
This book provides guidance on designing and conducting successful surveys using both traditional and online approaches.

Edwards, J. E., Thomas, M. D., Rosenfeld, P., & Booth-Kewley, S. (1997). *How to conduct organizational surveys: A step-by-step guide.* Thousand Oaks, Calif.: Sage.
This book covers exactly what you would expect: how to design, deploy, and analyze various types of surveys in organizations. It provides practical guidelines and worked examples to help the novice as well as the more experienced to fine-tune their survey skills.

Evaluation francophonie. Retrieved March 25, 2007, from http://www.evaluation.francophonie.org.
This site presents a collection of links to evaluation web sites. It aims to facilitate the evaluation community's networking and joint work with the French-speaking evaluation community.

Krueger, R. A., & Casey, M. A. (2000). *Focus groups: A practical guide for applied research* (3rd ed.). Thousand Oaks, Calif.: Sage.
This book provides a detailed step-by-step road map of how to design, prepare for, implement, analyze, and report on focus groups. It is useful for both novices and experienced evaluators.

Morgan, D. L. (1998). *The focus group guidebook.* Thousand Oaks, Calif.: Sage.
This is a useful introduction to using focus groups to collect qualitative data. The book describes the strengths and weaknesses of this technique, when to use it, what resources are needed, and how to use focus groups to engage stakeholders.

Payne, S. L. (1951). *The art of asking questions.* Princeton, N.J.: Princeton University Press.
This classic text provides practical suggestions on questions to be asked in surveys, interviews, and focus groups. Included is a checklist of 100 considerations that can be a useful tool.

Phillips, J. (Ed.) (1998). *Implementing evaluation systems and processes.* Alexandria, Va.: American Society for Training and Development.
This book contains 18 case studies from a cross-section of practitioners and organizations. Part 1 focuses on systematic evaluation practices. Part 2 presents specific techniques for assessing programs.

Russ-Eft, D. (2006). Communicating and reporting. In K. Hanmum, J. Martineau, & C. Reinelt (Eds.), *Handbook of leadership development evaluation.* San Francisco: Jossey-Bass.
This chapter examines issues related to communicating and reporting evaluation results specifically within an organizational context. It identifies some effective approaches to enhance the use of results.

Schonlau, M., Fricker, R., & Elliott, M. (2002). *Conducting research surveys via e-mail and the web.* Santa Monica, Calif.: RAND.
This book discusses the scope and limits of using e-mail and the web to do surveys. The authors offer many practical suggestions for designing and implementing Internet surveys most effectively.

Stadius, R. (1999). *More evaluation instruments (ASTD Trainers Toolkit).* Alexandria, Va.: American Society for Training and Development.
This publication contains sample evaluation instruments and articles on effective evaluation.

Torres, R. T., Preskill, H., & Piontek, M. (2005). *Evaluation strategies for communicating and reporting: Enhancing learning in organizations* (2nd ed.). Thousand Oaks, Calif.: Sage.
This text provides details on a variety of approaches to communicating and reporting to support evaluation use. It helps evaluators to determine and plan the most appropriate strategies for communicating and reporting to a variety of stakeholders.

Tufte, E. (2006). *Beautiful evidence.* Cheshire, Conn.: Graphics Press LLC.
This text focuses on the visual communication of information and discusses how to use graphics not merely to display data but to tell the underlying story.

Whitney, D., Cooperrider, D., Trosten-Bloom, A., & Kaplin, B. S. (2002). *Encyclopedia of positive questions: Using appreciative inquiry to bring out the best in your organization.* Euclid, Ohio: Lakeshore Communications.
This book provides questions that are central to the discovery phase of the appreciative inquiry process and that are key to bringing out the best in any organization. It is particularly useful when working with focus groups.

MANAGING THE EVALUATION

Bell, J. B. (2004). Managing evaluation projects step by step. In J. S. Wholey, H. P. Hatry, & K. E. Newcomer (Eds.), *Handbook of practical program evaluation* (2nd ed.). San Francisco: Jossey-Bass.
This chapter provides basic approaches to managing evaluation projects and includes topics related to clarifying the project, staffing, assignments and scheduling, monitoring progress, and product quality.

Beyerlein, M. M., Freedman, S., McGee, C., & Moran, L. (2002). *Beyond teams: Building the collaborative organization.* San Francisco: Pfeiffer.
This book focuses on developing collaborative organizational systems. Some of these ideas can be useful when trying to collaborate with evaluation team personnel and stakeholders.

Boulmetis, J., & Dutwin, P. (2005). *The ABCs of evaluation: Timeless techniques for program and project managers* (2nd ed.). San Francisco: Jossey-Bass.
This book covers many aspects in managing an evaluation, including how to deal with the multiple goals and objectives of the organization,

the staff, and the client. It contains cases and scenarios from various evaluation settings.

Fosberg, K., Mooz, H., & Cotterman, H. (2000). *Visualizing project management: A model for business and technical success.* New York: Wiley.
This book covers all aspects of project management, including project requirements, project planning, risks and opportunities, project control, corrective action, and project leadership.

Hoefling, T. (2001). *Working virtually: Managing people for successful virtual teams and organizations.* Sterling, Va.: Stylus.
This book provides useful guidelines for those managing virtual project teams, including teams located in different countries. An appendix includes a number of useful tools and checklists.

Kirkpatrick, D. L. (2006). *How to conduct productive meetings: Strategies, tips and tools to ensure that your next meeting is well planned and effective.* Alexandria, Va.: American Society for Training and Development.
This book provides practical tools and advice for anyone planning or facilitating a meeting. Legendary evaluation guru Donald Kirkpatrick offers advice to ensure that a meeting is necessary, the presentation is professional and effective, the participants contribute in constructive ways, and the outcome is measurable.

Moran, L., Musselwhite, E., & Zenger, J. H. (1996). *Keeping teams on track: What to do when the going gets rough.* Chicago: Irwin.
This book deals with problems that can arise with teams. It includes a series of tools and techniques that can be used to diagnose and solve some of those problems.

Phillips, J. P., Phillips, P. P., & Hodges, T. K. (2004). *Make training evaluation work.* Alexandria, Va.: American Society for Training and Development.
This book is designed to break through the organizational inertia facing many trainers and to show how to implement a fully functional evaluation program that is integrated throughout the learning process.

Zenger, J. H., Musselwhite, E., Hurson, K., & Perrin, C. (1994). *Leading teams: Mastering the new role.* Homewood, Ill.: Business One Irwin.
This book describes approaches to leading internal teams. It includes interviews with team leaders from various types of organizations.

APPENDIX

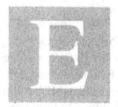

PROFESSIONAL ASSOCIATIONS FOR EVALUATORS

African Evaluation Association (http://www.afread.org)

American Evaluation Association (http://eval.org)

Aotearoa New Zealand Evaluation Association
(http://www.anzea.org.nz)

Australasian Evaluation Society (http://www.aes.asn.au)

Brazilian Evaluation Network (http://www.avaliabrasil.org.br)

Canadian Evaluation Society (http://www.evaluationcanada.ca)

Central American Evaluation Association (Contact Johanna Fernandez
for further information: johannaf@cariari.ucr.ac.cr)

Danish Evaluation Society (http://www.danskevalueringsselskab.dk)*

Dutch Evaluation Society (http://www.videnet.nl)*

European Evaluation Society (http://www.europeanevaluation.org)

Finnish Evaluation Society (http://www.finnishevaluationsociety.net)

French Evaluation Society (http://www.sfe.asso.fr)*

German Evaluation Society (http://www.degeval.de)*

International Organisation for Cooperation in Evaluation
(http://internationalevaluation.com)

International Program Evaluation Network (http://www.eval-net.org)*
Israeli Association for Program Evaluation (http://www.iape.org.il)*
Italian Evaluation Society (http://www.valutazione.it)*
Japan Evaluation Society (http://www.idcj.or.jp/JES)*
Latin American and Caribbean Programme for Strengthening the
    Regional Capacity for Monitoring and Evaluation of IFAD's Rural
    Poverty-Alleviation Projects (http://www.preval.org)
Malaysian Evaluation Society (http://www.mes.org.my)
Nigerien Monitoring and Evaluation Network
    (http://www.pnud.ne/rense/HOMEUK.html)
Polish Evaluation Society (http://www.pte.org.pl)*
Quebec Society for Program Evaluation (http://www.sqep.ca)*
Red de seguimiento, evaluacion y sistematization en América Latina y
    el Caribe (http://www.relacweb.org)*
South African Evaluation Network
    (http://www.afrea.org/webs/southafrica)
South African Monitoring and Evaluation Association
    (http://www.samea.org.za)
Spanish Public Policy Evaluation Society
    (http://www.sociedadevaluacion.org)*
Sri Lanka Evaluation Association (http://www.nsf.ac.lk/sleva)
Swedish Evaluation Society (http://www.statskontoret.se)*
Swiss Evaluation Society (http://www.seval.ch/en)
Uganda Evaluation Association
    (http://institutions.africadatabase.org/data/i115507.html)
United Kingdom Evaluation Society (http://www.evaluation.org.uk)
Washington Research Evaluation Network (http://www.wren-network.net)

*Web site offers limited information in English.

REFERENCES

Academy of Human Resource Development (1999). *Standards on ethics and integrity.* Baton Rouge, La.: Academy of Human Resource Development. Retrieved February 9, 2003, from http://www.ahrd.org/publications/.

African Evaluation Association (2002). *The African evaluation guidelines: 2002.* Retrieved January 11, 2005, from http://www.afrea.org/content/index.cfm?navID=5&itemID=204.

Altschuld, J. W., Engle, M., Cullen, C., Kim, I., & Mace, B. R. (1994). The 1994 directory of evaluation training programs. In J. W. Altschuld & M. Engle (Eds.), *The preparation of professional evaluators: Issues, perspectives, and programs.* New Directions for Program Evaluation, No. 62, pp. 71–94. San Francisco: Jossey-Bass.

American Evaluation Association (1995). Guiding principles for evaluators. In W. R. Shadish, D. L. Newman, M. A. Scheirer, & C. Wye (Eds.), *Guiding principles for evaluators.* New Directions for Program Evaluation, No. 66. San Francisco: Jossey-Bass.

American Evaluation Association (2004, July). *Guiding principles for evaluators.* Retrieved January 11, 2005, from http://www.eval.org/Publications/GuidingPrinciples.asp.

Australasian Evaluation Society (n.d.). *Code of ethics.* Retrieved December 23, 2006, from http://www.aes.asn.au.

Australasian Evaluation Society (2006, July). *Guidelines for the ethical conduct of evaluations.* Retrieved December 23, 2006, from http://www.aes.asn.au.

Bamberger, M., Rugh, J., & Mabry, L. (2006). *RealWorld evaluation: Working under budget, time, data, and political constraints.* Thousand Oaks, Calif.: Sage.

Bartel, A. P. (1997). Return-on-investment. In L. J. Bassi & D. Russ-Eft (Eds.), *What works: Assessment, development, and measurement.* Alexandria, Va.: American Society for Training and Development.

Basarab, D. J., Sr., & Root, D. K. (1992). *The training evaluation process.* Boston: Kluwer.

Beywl, W., & Taut, S. (Trans.) (2001, February). Summary of evaluation standards, presented by the German Evaluation Society (DeGEval-Standards). Los Angeles. Retrieved September 13, 2007, from http://www.degeval.de/index.php?class=Calimero_Webpage&id=9023.

Bloom, B. S., Engelhart, M. D., Furst, E. J., Hill, W. H., & Krathwohl, D. R. (1956). *Taxonomy of educational objectives: Handbook I. Cognitive domain.* New York: David McKay.

Briggs, L. (1977). *Instructional design: Principles and applications.* Englewood Cliffs, N.J.: Educational Technology Publications.

Brinkerhoff, R. O. (1988). An integrated evaluation model for HRD. *Training and Development Journal, 42*(2), 66–68.

Brinkerhoff, R. O. (1989). *Achieving results from training.* San Francisco: Jossey-Bass.

Brinkerhoff, R. O. (2003). *The success case method: Find out quickly what's working and what's not.* San Francisco: Berrett-Koehler.

Brinkerhoff, R. O. (2005). The success case method: A strategic evaluation approach to increasing the value and effect of training. In G. G. Wang & D. R. Spitzer (Eds.), Advances in HRD measurement and evaluation: Theory and practice. *Advances in Developing Human Resources, 7*(1), pp. 86–101. Thousand Oaks, Calif.: Sage.

Brinkerhoff, R. O. (2006). *Telling training's story: Evaluation made simple, credible, and effective.* San Francisco: Berrett-Koehler.

Brinkerhoff, R. O., & Gill, S. J. (1994). *The learning alliance: Systems thinking in human resource development.* San Francisco: Jossey-Bass.

Burns, J. Z., Russ-Eft, D., & Wright, H. F. (2001). Codes of ethics and enforcement of ethical conduct: A review of other organizations and implications for AHRD. In O. Aliaga (Ed.), *Academy of Human Resource Development: 2001 Conference Proceedings, 1,* pp. 213–220.

Buros Institute; Murphy, L. L., Plake, B. S., & Spies, R. A. (2006). *Tests in print.* Lincoln, Neb.: Buros Institute of Mental Measurements.

Buros Institute; Spies, R. A., Plake, B. S., Geisinger, K. F., & Carlson, J. F. (2007). *The seventeenth mental measurement yearbook.* Buros mental measurement yearbooks. Lincoln, Neb.: Buros Institute of Mental Measurements.

Bushnell, D. S. (1990). Input, process, output: A model for evaluating training. *Training and Development Journal, 42*(3), 41–43.

Cambridge University Press (2007). Profession. In *Cambridge Dictionaries Online.* Retrieved March 23, 2007, from http://dictionary.cambridge.org.

Canadian Evaluation Society (1996). *CES guidelines for ethical conduct.* Retrieved May 6, 2003, from http://www.evaluationcanada.ca/site.cgi?s=5&ss+4&_lang=an.

Catano, V. (1998). *Competencies: A review of the literature and bibliography. National standards for human resources professionals.* Development phase, Phase 1. Canadian Council of Human Resources Association/Conseil canadien des associations en resources humaines. Retrieved September 13, 2007, from http://www.chrpcanada.com/en/phaseIreport/appendix.asp.

Deutsche Gesellschaft für Evaluation (DeGEval) (2001, October 4). *Standards für evaluation.* Retrieved May 6, 2003, from http://www.degeval.de/index.php?class=Calimero_Webpage&id=9023.

Dick, W. O., Carey, L., & Carey, J. O. (2004). *Systematic design of instruction* (6th ed.). Boston: Allyn & Bacon.

Dick, W., Watson, K., & Kaufman, R. (1981). Deriving competencies: Consensus versus model building. *Educational Researcher, 10*(8), 5–10.

Donaldson, S. I., & Christie, C. A. (2006). Emerging career opportunities in the transdiscipline of evaluation science. In S. I. Donaldson, D. E. Berger, & K. Pezdek (Eds.), *Applied psychology: New frontiers and rewarding careers*, pp. 243–259. Mahwah, N.J.: Lawrence Erlbaum Associates.

Engle, M., Altschuld, J. W., & Kim, Y.-C. (2006). 2002 survey of evaluation preparation programs in universities: An update of the 1992 American Evaluation Association sponsored study. *American Journal of Evaluation, 27*(3), 353–359.

Erickson, P. R. (1990). Evaluating training results. *Training and Development Journal, 44*(1), 57–59.

Fitzpatrick, J. L., Sanders, J. R., & Worthen, B. R. (2004). *Program evaluation: Alternative approaches and practical guidelines* (3rd ed.). Boston: Pearson Education.

Flanagan, J. C. (1949). A new approach to evaluating personnel. *Personnel, 26,* 35–42.

Flanagan, J. C. (1954). The critical incident technique. *Psychological Bulletin, 51*(4), 327–358.

Foxon, M. J. (1994). A process approach to transfer of training. Part 2: Using action planning to facilitate the transfer of training. *Australian Journal of Educational Technology, 10*(1), 1–18.

Foxon, M., Richey, R. C., Roberts, R. C., & Spannaus, T. (2003). *Training manager competencies: The standards* (3rd ed.). Syracuse, N.Y.: ERIC Clearinghouse on Information and Technology.

Gates, S. (2005). *Measuring more than efficiency.* Report No. R-1356–04-RR. New York: Conference Board.

Ghere, G., King, J. A., Stevahn, L., & Minnema, J. (2006). A professional development unit for reflecting on program evaluator competencies. *American Journal of Evaluation, 27*(1), 108–123.

Guba, E. G., & Lincoln, Y. S. (1981). *Effective evaluations.* San Francisco: Jossey-Bass.

Hale, J. (2000). *Performance-based certification: How to design a valid, defensible, cost-effective program.* San Francisco: Jossey-Bass/Pfeiffer.

Hamblin, A. C. (1974). *Evaluation and control of training.* London: McGraw-Hill.

Hendry, I., & Maggio, E. (1996, May). Tracking success: Is competency-based human resources management an effective strategy or simply flavour of the month? *Benefits Canada, 20,* 71.

Hilbert, J., Preskill, H., & Russ-Eft, D. (1997). Evaluating training. In L. J. Bassi & D. Russ-Eft (Eds.), *What works: Assessment, development, and measurement,* pp. 109–150. Alexandria, Va.: American Society for Training and Development.

Holton, E. F., III. (1996). The flawed four-level evaluation model. *Human Resource Development Quarterly, 7*(1), 5–21.

Holton, E. F., III. (2005). Holton's evaluation model: New evidence and construct elaboration. In G. G. Wang & D. R. Spitzer (Eds.), *Advances in HRD measurement and evaluation: Theory and practice. Advances in Developing Human Resources, 7*(1), 37–54. Thousand Oaks, Calif.: Sage.

Hooghiemstra, T. (1992). Integrated management of human resources. In A. Mitrani, M. Dalziel, & D. Fitt (Eds.), *Competency based human resource management,* pp. 17–46. London: Kogan Page.

HR Guide to the Internet (http://www.hr-guide.com/compensation.htm). Integrating competencies into HR programs. Retrieved September 10, 2007, from http://www.hr-guide.com/data/G480.htm.

Hurteau, M. (1993). *Reflections on a code of ethics.* Discussion paper presented to the National Council of the Canadian Evaluation Society, Banff, Canada.

International Board of Standards for Training, Performance, and Instruction (1993, 2003). *Instructor competencies.* Retrieved March 21, 2007, from http://www.ibstpi.org/downloads/InstructorCompetencies.pdf.

Joint Committee on Educational and Psychological Tests (American Educational Research Association, American Psychological Association, and National Council on Measurement in Education.) (1999). *Standards for educational and psychological testing.* Washington, D.C.: Author.

Joint Committee on Educational and Psychological Tests (1999). *Standards for educational and psychological testing.* Washington, D.C.: American Educational Research Association.

Joint Committee on Standards for Educational Evaluation (1981). *Standards for evaluations of educational programs, projects, and materials.* New York: McGraw-Hill.

Joint Committee on Standards for Educational Evaluation (1994). *The program evaluation standards* (2nd ed.). Thousand Oaks, Calif.: Sage.

Kaufman, R., & Keller, J. M. (1994). Levels of evaluation: Beyond Kirkpatrick. *Human Resource Development Quarterly, 5*(4), 371–380.

Kaufman, R., Keller, J., & Watkins, R. (1995). What works and what doesn't: Evaluation beyond Kirkpatrick. *Performance and Instruction, 35*(2), 8–12.

Keith, G. (2003, June). The Canadian Evaluation Society (CES) experience in developing standards for evaluation and ethical issues. Paper presented at the 5th European conference on the Evaluation of Structural Funds, Budapest, Hungary. Retrieved December 22, 2006, from http://evaluationcanada.ca/distribution/20030626_keith_gwen.pdf.

Kierstead, J. (1998). Competencies and KSAOs. Research Directorate. Policy, Research and Communications Branch. Public Service Commission of Canada. Human resources management agency of Canada. Retrieved September 13, 2007, from http://www.psagency-agencefp.gc.ca/research/personnel/comp_ksao_e.pdf.

King, J. A., Stevahn, L., Ghere, G., & Minnema, J. (2001). Toward a taxonomy of essential evaluator competencies. *American Journal of Evaluation, 22,* 229–247.

Kirkpatrick, D. L. (1959a, November). Techniques for evaluating programs. *Journal of the American Society of Training Directors (Training and Development Journal), 13*(11), 3–9.

Kirkpatrick, D. L. (1959b, December). Techniques for evaluating programs-Part 2: Learning. *Journal of the American Society of Training Directors (Training and Development Journal), 13*(12), 21–26.

Kirkpatrick, D. L. (1960a, January). Techniques for evaluating programs-Part 3: Behavior. *Journal of the American Society of Training Directors (Training and Development Journal), 14*(1), 13–18.

Kirkpatrick, D. L. (1960b, January). Techniques for evaluating programs-Part 4: Results. *Journal of the American Society of Training Directors (Training and Development Journal), 14*(1), 28–32.

Kirkpatrick, D. L. (1994). *Evaluating training programs: The four levels.* San Francisco: Berrett-Koehler.

Klein, A. L. (1996). Validity and reliability for competency-based systems: Reducing litigation risks. *Compensation and Benefits Review, 28,* 31–37.

Klein, J. D., Spector, J. M., Grabowski, B., & de la Teja, I. (2004). *Instructor competencies: Standards for face-to-face, online, and blended settings.* Greenwich, Conn.: Information Age.

Klemp, G. O. (1980). *The assessment of occupational competence.* Washington, D.C.: Report to the National Institute of Education.

Kraiger, K., Ford, J. K., & Salas, E. (1993). Application of cognitive, skill-based, and affective theories of learning outcomes to new methods of training evaluation. *Journal of Applied Psychology, 78*(2), 311–328.

Le Boterf, G. (2001). *Construire les competences individuelles et collectives.* Paris: Editions d'Organisation.

Lincoln, R. E., & Dunet, D. O. (1995). Training efficiency and effectiveness model (TEEM). *Performance and Instruction, 34*(3), 40–47.

Lucia, D., & Lepsinger, R. (1999). *The art and science of competency models: Pinpointing critical success factors in organizations.* San Francisco: Jossey-Bass/Pfeiffer.

McClelland, D. A. (1973). Testing for competence rather than for intelligence. *American Psychologist, 28*(1), 1–14.

McDavid, J. C., & Hawthorn, L. R. (2006). *Program evaluation and performance measurement: An introduction to practice.* Thousand Oaks, Calif.: Sage.

McLagan, P. (1989). Models for HRD practice. *Training and Development, 43*(9), 49–59.

McLagan, P. A. (1997). Competencies: The next generation. *Training and Development, 51*(5), 40–47. ERIC Document Reproduction Service No. EJ 543 935.

Mager, R. F. (1962). *Preparing instructional objectives.* Palo Alto, Calif.: Fearon Press.

Marrelli, A. F. (1998). An introduction to competency analysis and modeling. *Performance Improvement, 37*(5), 8–17.

National Center for O*NET Development (n.d.). Occupational Information Network Resource Center (O*NET). Retrieved September 10, 2007, from http://www.onetcenter.org/.

Newman, C., & Brown, R. (1996). *Applied ethics for program evaluation.* Thousand Oaks, Calif.: Sage.

Owen, J. M., & Rogers, P. J. (1999). *Program evaluation: Forms and approaches.* London: Sage.

Parry, S. B. (1998, June). Just what is a competency? (and, why should you care?) *Training, 35*(6), 58–64.

Patton, M. Q. (1997). *Utilization-focused evaluation: The new century text.* Thousand Oaks, Calif.: Sage.

Phillips, J. J. (1997a). *Return on investment in training and performance improvement programs.* Houston: Gulf.

Phillips, J. J., (1997b). *Handbook of training evaluation and measurement methods* (3rd ed.). Houston: Gulf.

Phillips, J. J., & Phillips, P. P. (2005). *ROI at work.* Alexandria, Va.: American Society for Training and Development.

Phillips, P. P., & Phillips, J. J. (2006). *Return on investment (ROI) basics.* Alexandria, Va.: American Society for Training and Development.

Preskill, H., & Russ-Eft, D. (2003). A framework for reframing HRD evaluation practice and research. In A. M. Gilley, L. Bierema, & J. Callahan (Eds.), *Critical issues in HRD,* pp. 199–257. Cambridge, Mass.: Perseus.

Preskill, H., & Russ-Eft, D. (2005). *Building evaluation capacity: 72 activities for teaching and training.* Thousand Oaks, Calif.: Sage.

Richey, R. C. (1992). *Designing instruction for the adult learner.* London: Kogan Page.

Richey, R. C. (2002). The ibstpi competency standards: Development, definition, and use. In M. A. Fitzgerald, M. Orey, & R. M. Branch (Eds.), *Educational media and technology yearbook (Vol. 27),* pp. 111–119. Englewood, Colo.: Greenwood.

Richey, R. C., Fields, D. C., & Foxon, M. (2001). *Instructional design competencies: The standards.* Syracuse, N.Y.: ERIC Clearinghouse on Information and Technology.

Rossi, P. H., Freeman, H. E., & Lipsey, M. W. (1999). *Evaluation: A systematic approach* (6th ed.). Thousand Oaks, Calif.: Sage.

Rossi, P. H., Lipsey, M. W., & Freeman, H. E. (2003). *Evaluation: A systematic approach* (7th ed.), Thousand Oaks, Calif.: Sage.

Rothwell, W. J. (1996). *ASTD models for human performance improvement: Roles, competencies, and outputs.* Alexandria, Va.: American Society for Training and Development.

Rowe, C. (1995). Clarifying the use of competence and competency models in recruitment, assessment, and staff development. *Industrial and Commercial Training, 27,* 12–17.

Ruona, W.E.A., & Rusaw, A. C. (2001). The role of codes of ethics in the human resource development. *Academy of Human Resource Development: 2001 Conference Proceedings, 1,* 221–228.

Russ-Eft, D. (1995). Defining competencies: A critique. (Editorial). *Human Resource Development Quarterly, 6,* 329–335.

Russ-Eft, D. (2004a). Customer service competencies: A global look. *Human Resource Development International, 7,* 211–231.

Russ-Eft, D. (2004b). Ethics in a global world: An oxymoron? *Evaluation and Program Planning, 27,* 349–356.

Russ-Eft, D. (2004c). In search of ethics and integrity in human resource development. In J. Woodall, M. Lee, & J. McGoldrick (Eds.), *New frontiers in human resource development,* pp. 43–57. London: Routledge.

Russ-Eft, D., & Preskill, H. (2001). *Evaluation in organizations: A systematic approach to enhancing learning, performance, and change.* Cambridge, Mass.; Perseus.

Russ-Eft, D., & Preskill, H. (2005). In search of the holy grail: ROI evaluation in HRD. In G. G. Wang & D. R. Spitzer (Eds.), *Advances in HRD measurement and evaluation: Theory and practice. Advances in Developing Human Resources, 7*(1), 71–85. Thousand Oaks, Calif.: Sage.

Scriven, M. (2003). Evaluation in the new millennium: The transdisciplinary vision. In S. I. Donaldson & M. Scriven (Eds.), *Evaluating social programs and problems: Vision for the new millennium,* pp. 19–42. Mahwah, N.J.: Lawrence Erlbaum.

Seels, B. B., & Richey, R. C. (1994). *Instructional technology: The definitions and domains of the field.* Washington, D.C.: Association for Educational Communications and Technology.

Smith, M. F. (1999). Should AEA begin a process for restricting membership in the profession of evaluation? *American Journal of Evaluation, 20,* 521–531.

Spencer, L. M., & Spencer, S. M. (1993). *Competence at work: Models for superior performance.* New York: Wiley.

Stephenson, J., & Raven, J. (Eds.), (2001). *Competence in the learning society.* New York: Lang.

Stevahn, L., King, J. A., Ghere, G., & Minnema, J. (2005). Establishing essential competencies for evaluators. *American Journal of Evaluation, 26*(1), 43–59.

Stevahn, L., King, J. A., Ghere, G., & Minnema, J. (2006). Evaluator competencies in university-based evaluation training programs. *Canadian Journal of Program Evaluation, 20*(1), 101–123.

Stufflebeam, D. L. (1983). The CIPP model for program evaluation. Chap. 7. In G. F. Madaus, M. Scriven, & D. L. Stufflebeam (Eds.), *Evaluation models,* pp. 117–141. Boston: Kluwer-Nijhoff.

Stufflebeam, D. L. (2000). The CIPP model for evaluation. Chap. 16. In D. L. Stufflebeam, G. F. Madaus, & T. Kellaghan (Eds.), *Evaluation models* (2nd ed.). Boston: Kluwer Academic.

Swanson, R. A., & Holton, E. F. (1999). *Results: How to assess performance, learning, and perceptions in organizations.* San Francisco: Berrett-Koehler.

Swanson, R. A., & Sleezer, C. M. (1987). Training effectiveness evaluation. *Journal of European Industrial Training, 11*(4), 7–16.

Taylor, P., Russ-Eft, D., & Chan, D. (2005). The effectiveness of behavior modeling training across settings and features of study design. *Journal of Applied Psychology, 90,* 692–709.

Toolsema, B. (2003). Werken met compententies. Naar een instrument voor de identificatie van competenties. Doctoral dissertation, Twente University, Netherlands.

Torres, R. T., Preskill, H., & Piontek, M. E. (2005). *Evaluation strategies for communicating and reporting: Enhancing learning in organizations* (2nd ed.). Thousand Oaks, Calif.: Sage.

Tyler, R. (1935). Evaluation: A challenge to progressive education. *Educational Research Bulletin, 14,* 9–16.

Van Merriënboer, J.J.G., Van der Klink, M. R., & Hendriks, M. (2002). *Competenties: Van complicaties tot compromis. Een studie in opdracht van de onderwijsraad* [Competencies: from complications towards a compromise–A study for the National Educational Council]. The Hague, Netherlands: Onderwijsraad.

Wang, G. G., & Spitzer, D. R. (Eds.), (2005). *Advances in HRD measurement and evaluation: Theory and practice. Advances in Developing Human Resources, 7*(1). Thousand Oaks, Calif.: Sage.

Weiss, C. H. (1987). Where politics and evaluation research meet. In D. J. Palumbo (Ed.), *The politics of program evaluation.* Newbury Park, Calif.: Sage.

Wholey, J. S. (1975). Evaluation: When is it really needed? *Evaluation Magazine, 2*(2).

Wholey, J. S. (1976). *A methodology for planning and conducting project impact evaluation in UNESCO fields.* Washington, D.C.: Urban Institute.

Wholey, J. S. (1979). *Evaluation: Promise and performance.* Washington, D.C.: Urban Institute.

Woodruff, C. (1991). Competent by any other name. *Personnel Management, 23,* 30–33.

Worthen, B. R., & Sanders, J. R. (1991). The changing face of educational evaluation. *Theory into Practice, 30,* 3–12.

Young, J. I., & Van Mondfrans, A. P. (1972). Psychological implications of competency-based education. *Educational Technology, 12*(11), 15–18.

Zorzi, R., McGuire, M., & Perrin, B. (2002, October). Canadian Evaluation Society project in support of advocacy and professional development: Evaluation benefits, outputs, and knowledge elements. Toronto, Canada: Zorzi & Associates. Retrieved December 22, 2006, from http://evaluationcanada.ca/distribution/200210_zorzi_e.pdf.

INDEX